I0481674

"As a result of a work injury, I searched for 20 years to find some kind of relief for pain that had plagued my life. As a result of Dr. Ennis's self-hypnosis, I was able to take control of my life again and put pain in its spot. The strategies and techniques that are taught by the doctor are very easy and straightforward to follow. With a little bit of practice virtually anyone can benefit from this."

—Bob Hodgins, injured worker

"Learning self-hypnosis has brought about a significant and appreciable change in my quality of life. With empathy and compassion for the chronic pain sufferer, Dr. Ennis affably and candidly teaches hypnotherapy program participants an understandable and relatable way to perform unique pain control methods using self-hypnosis. The 10-week hypnotherapy program was a personal success and is something I'd recommend to other chronic pain sufferers. This teaching is an excellent tool for anyone with chronic pain!"

—Kezia Smykaluk, participant,
10-week Hypnotherapy Program

"Sometimes our best teachers in life are those who have been in our shoes, and Dr. Ennis is one of the best examples of that. He has been a source of inspiration for me when pain made me want to give up. After taking his course on hypnotherapy for pain management, I was finally able to break free from addiction to opiates for pain relief. If you are suffering chronic pain and are frustrated at the lack of results from various treatments, or if you are tired of relying on pain killers, this book could be the life changer you been looking for."

—Paul D. Carr, patient

"Dr. Ennis shares his personal experiences as a patient and professional insights as a pain expert. This is presented in a thoughtful and engaging manner. His perspective related to the role of hypnotherapy will be of interest to patients and physicians alike."

—Nesathurai Shanker, MD, Chief Division of
Physical Medicine and Rehabilitation, Department
of Medicine, Hamilton Health Sciences

"Drawing on his personal and clinical experiences, Dr. Ennis has produced an easy-to-read, practical, and very helpful guide for anyone living with chronic pain. Avoiding jargon, he walks the reader through commonly employed treatment approaches and highlights things anyone can take to manage their own care. In particular, he emphasizes the role of self-hypnosis as a simple and effective way for a person to master their pain and minimize its effect on their life, with a step-by-step guide as to how to use it. This is a very valuable resource for anyone with chronic pain."

—Nick Kates, MD, Chair and Professor, Psychiatry and
Behavioural Neurosciences, McMaster University

*I dedicate this book to my wife, Gilda. Without her,
I would never have been able to face the many challenges
I have, nor would I have become a physician, psychiatrist,
and pain specialist. Without her, this book would never
have been written. She truly is "Everything" to me.
"Everything" is the title of a song I wrote for Gilda.
If you would like to hear it you can find it at:
https://youtu.be/9lN9TtnpU44*

Contents

Acknowledgments

I n a life peppered by many challenges, there are people who have helped me move forward. Without them, my life would have been very different. My father, David, was a very quiet, kind, soft-spoken man who did his best to be there for me. My mother, Rita, could make things challenging but she did push me forward to find the best that I have to offer, even under adversity. Both of them are gone now. My father-in-law, Irving, always liked to have an argument with me, and I always gave him one. He helped me sharpen my wits but I always admired his own bravery in managing terrible adversity. Irving is also gone. My mother-in-law, Faye, is at the end of her days now. She always showed me kindness and patience except when I was about 16 and she wanted me to leave her home because it was after 12:00 p.m. She threw her shoes down the stairs. I'm sure that is the most aggressive thing she ever did. She and Irving gave me my lovely wife, Gilda.

Together Gilda and I have four wonderful sons, Jesse, Daniel, Jonathan, and Jamie. I remember telling Gilda when they were very young, "Who needs a psychotherapist?" Just watch and listen to your kids. They will tell you and show you everything you need to work on. Well, they still keep telling and showing me and I keep learning. Thank you, guys. They have wonderful wives, my daughters-in-law, Nikki and Kate. Without daughters-in-law I would never have had the experience of daughters. They definitely hug differently than guys. Of course there are my two grand-sons, Hudson and Gavin, from Jesse and Nikki. Now my psychotherapy goes even deeper. All of you have made my life worthwhile. You give me a reason to rise above the pain that life can throw at us.

Thank you to two friends, Glenn and Richard, one of whom was the very first editor of my first draft for this book. As I tell patients who, by the time they see me, feel isolated and alone, if you have one close friend that is amazing. If you have two, that is a miracle. You know your friends are close if you can call them in the middle of the night and ask for help—and they don't ask why. These two gentlemen have been with me through thick and thin since my early twenties. There is nothing they wouldn't do for me and there is nothing I would not do for them. Glenn is the kindest of souls and Richard is the most loyal and toughest guy I know. They maintain my faith in humanity and help me believe that tomorrow will be better.

Someone like me has seen many health care providers. I have either worked with them or have seen them as a patient. The following people have enriched my life as a professional, a teacher, and a person. They have never looked at me as less because of my own physical challenges and have always expected me to give the best that I have. Special thanks to Dr. Susan Goodwin, the neurologist on call the very first night I was admitted to the hospital almost 30 years ago. I was very sick, but she calmed me down and does so every time I see her. When I met Dr. John Kelton, who became the Dean of McMaster University's Medical Program, I was very sick, unable to stand up independently. He was the first person to offer me plasmapharesis to treat the horrible disease that has changed my life. He came in on weekends, and he gave me confidence that things would work out. Dr. Drew Bednar is an incredible orthopaedic surgeon who has twice helped me walk and I will always be grateful to him. Dr. Brian Steele once mentioned just in passing that I might want to try IgG, a type of antibody therapy, instead of plasmapharesis. It made managing my disease so much easier. Thank you to Dr. Walter Bobechko, who is no longer with us and was the very first orthopaedic surgeon I saw who tried to fix my right knee, and to Dr. Ezra Silverstein, who fixed my left. Without them, I would have had a lot of trouble walking. Both Dr. Herbert Von Schroder and Dr. Carolyn Levis have done several surgeries on my hands, which have allowed me to keep painting, building, and playing guitar. I also want to thank Dr. Bobby Shayegan and Dr. Himansu Lukka, both of whom are now doing their best to keep me alive. Dr. Neil Finnie is the primary care physician's physician. I had the pleasure of consulting in his office for many years and had the chance of seeing all that a GP can be. Because of that, I found Dr. David Johns, a trainee of Dr. Finnie who has been my primary care physician through thick and thin. I suppose I'm one of the worst patients you can get. I have uncommon diseases and I probably know more about them than my doctor does. Dr. Johns has always treated me with respect and compassion and has always brought something helpful to the table. Thank you to Dr. Susan Waserman. She has been my immunologist for over 25 years and has managed to keep me going all this time. She is generous with her expertise, and humanity. Thank you to all of these wonderful clinicians.

My career in pain management began before I finished my residency in psychiatry. In 1992 Gilda and I had taken our three sons to New Zealand. The boys were eight, six, and four. Jamie, our youngest, was still a twinkle in our eyes. I did a rotation in Child Psychiatry in Christchurch. At that time I was planning on being a child psychiatrist. By the time we got home, I had a serious relapse of my immune disease. At this time Gilda was a physiotherapist in the only multidisciplinary pain program in the area. She and her colleagues (most of whom are still friends) got together and decided I should do a rotation in pain management. I was quite ill but I couldn't sit at home. The longer I did that, the longer it would be before I finished my residency. I met with the head of the program, Dr. Eldon Tunks. He knew I was sick and he knew I had chronic pain from all my surgeries. Whenever I met a supervisor, I was always very honest about what I could do. I explained to him I was not 100 percent at that time. He said, "Come and do what you can." Might seem reasonable to you, but as resident, his statement was unheard of. Typically, supervisors are more like somewhat benign vampires. In exchange for teaching of variable quality, they will suck all the life energy you have for the purpose of delivering service to patients. "Do what you can" was a real shock to me. I did come and I did do what I could. I got stronger over time. More importantly, I discovered that my own illness and pain had a purpose. I understood these patients. It helped to make sense of my own suffering and I was hooked. I will always be grateful to Dr. Tunks for giving an impaired person a chance. It truly changed my life.

I have treated patients for over 30 years and been in the business of pain management for 25. I have run my own programs for close to 20 years. Most of my colleagues in my pain program started working with me when I was introduced to pain management as a resident in 1992. They are still with me to this day: Martha, Debbie, Sharon, Gilda (of course), Mike, and Michelle. It has been an honour for me to work with these people. They make me look good every day and I learn something from them every time I see them. They have also helped me deal with my own issues through their support, respect, and kindness. Thank you.

My office manager and support for over 20 years, Susan Carreau, has watched my practice change. She has seen programs grow and develop. She has seen me through the best of times and the worst of times. Who knew when she walked into my office 20 years ago that I had found not only an indispensible resource who helps me look better to the world around me every day, but also a good friend to Gilda and me? Susan and her husband, Dan, as well as her wonderful daughter and sons, have been there when the chips were down. Who could ask for more?

Ann Brodie helped Gilda and me set up the Ennis Endowment Fund (described in more detail at the end of this book). This is a fund designed to get residents of medicine interested in chronic pain management. It is our hope that this fund will help to find future pain specialists. Ann has put her heart and soul into this project and it is greatly appreciated. I knew from the moment I first met her that we would be friends. When we met her husband and artist, Frank, bonus. How lucky can you get.

There are a host of friends that have tried their best to pick me up when I'm down. Angela and Elani I met when I was a resident in pain management and they are still close friends. If I could find a way, I would steal them both for my own pain program. There are also many friends of Gilda and other people who one way or another have enriched my life. If I have not named you here, know that you are not forgotten.

I would be remiss if I did not thank my primary editor, Sarah Scott of Barlow Publishing. I met Sarah because of her sister Martha. Martha is the occupational therapist in my pain program and I have worked with her, and been her friend, for close to 30 years. This project was born at my first meeting with Sarah at a party at Martha's house. (I'm sure Martha set this up.) Sarah has had to work with me through the ups and downs of my health and my incredibly demanding nature. She stuck with it. Without her willingness to stick with it, this book would never have been in your hands now.

Last, I would like to acknowledge all those patients whom I have treated over the decades of my career that have taught me something. Some of them have volunteered in my programs for many years. As a physician I get a great deal out of my patients. I hope I give as much as I get. I have seen incredible bravery over the years that I can only admire and learn from.

To all of these people, a heart felt thank you.

Introduction

The greatest evil is physical pain.
—Saint Augustine
(354–430 BCE)

I am the kind of patient who challenges most physicians. I have chronic pain, the kind of pain that will never go away. It's all over my body. My back has hurt badly since I was a teenager, and it still hurts after a half dozen surgeries. I also have a strange syndrome you see in circus contortionists, which has led to another dozen orthopedic surgeries. That's not all. I have a weird immunologic disease resulting in episodic loss of muscle power and patchy burning pain all over my body. I am in pain every day, all day.

It has been a struggle at times to get my treating physicians to understand what is happening to me and how this pain is doing its best to destroy my life. Some doctors get it, and I have continued to see them for almost 30 years. Unfortunately, most physicians have trouble understanding what it is like to have chronic pain all day, every day. One physician actually suggested that my pain was in my mind. When he said that, I thought, Okay, if that is true, I can stop all the poisonous medications I have to take. He was wrong. Three months later, the disease that was supposed to be in my mind came back with a vengeance. I felt pain ripping down my right leg, and soon after, I lost the use of that leg. I was measured for a wheelchair and told by another sensitive physician that this would be it for the rest of my life. Well, he was wrong too.

Having chronic pain can make me feel helpless, and even hopeless at times. It frustrates me because I am not just a patient; I am a medical doctor. I trained as a psychiatrist, and trained a lot more to become a specialist in treating chronic pain. I have made a 25-year career as a specialist in chronic pain. So I'm in the unusual position of seeing chronic pain from both sides—as a patient who lives it every day, and as a doctor who is struggling to understand this mysterious and all too common problem. Having chronic pain myself makes the job of doctor a little easier in one respect, though. When patients come to see me with a complaint about chronic pain, I never question them. I never say it's all in their head. Why would I? The vast majority of patients would not tell me they have pain if they didn't. Unfortunately, some of my colleagues in the medical profession do not think this way. I suspect it's because they do not have a solid understanding of chronic pain. Chronic pain is not a major topic in the undergraduate medical curriculum. In fact, at the medical school that I'm associated with, the only instruction students got on the topic of chronic pain was a two-hour lecture from me. Honest. Even then, I noticed that most of the students were busy on their devices during my lecture, so I stopped. That was five years ago. Perhaps it has changed since then.

Pain relief is often left behind the other major advances of medicine. For patients, this can become a huge gap in their medical care. Although we live in a world filled with amazing medical breakthroughs, the millions of patients worldwide with chronic pain have not been the recipients of these gifts. In fact, the mainstay of medical management of chronic pain is a medication that has been in use for over 5,000 years: opioids, which include morphine and its derivatives. The prescription of this ancient remedy has increased exponentially over the last 20 years. Since this remedy is prescribed by physicians, you might think it has helped people to lead relatively normal lives. Unfortunately, for the most part, this is not the case. Although opioids can help reduce pain, they do not remove it. In fact, opioids are less effective for treating chronic pain than many physicians believe, and they do not help people function better. They do cause a plethora of terrible and even deadly side effects, such as addiction to opioids, which has increased dramatically over the past decade. Deaths due to opioids for pain control have soared. In 2014 alone,

14,000 Americans and an estimated 2,000 Canadians died of opioids prescribed by doctors.

It's a doctor-prescribed opioid epidemic, and, as I wrote this book, authorities were finally taking the first steps to curb the problem. In 2016, the Centers for Disease Control (CDC) took action to curb the amount of opioids that doctors were prescribing. The CDC advised clinicians to start with "the lowest effective dosage" and significantly reduced the recommended upper limit to 90 milligram equivalents of morphine per day. Canada produced its guidelines in 2017. Guideline number 6 states, "We recommend restricting the prescribed dose to less than 90 mg morphine equivalents daily rather than no upper limit or a higher limit on dosing." This is considered a strong recommendation, meaning there is significant data to support the statement. The seventh recommendation states: "For patients with chronic noncancer pain who are beginning opioid therapy, we suggest restricting the prescribed dose to less than 50 mg morphine equivalents daily." This is a weak recommendation. So, in summary, the Canadian guideline indicates that in a patient with no other issues outside of chronic pain they should be treated with no more than 50 mg of morphine equivalent and if necessary go up to a maximum of 90 mg.

This changes the picture for people with chronic pain: doctors are not going to be prescribing such high doses of opioids to help manage chronic pain as they have in the past. Now the problem for doctors is this: If we can't prescribe high doses of opioids, what do we tell our patients with chronic pain? What do we do? How will we live a good life without the medication we would like to believe will help us?

From my own experience, I know that if you have chronic pain you have a very tough choice to make. Are you going to let the pain run your life? Are you going to let yourself be burned at the stake by your pain, and as the fire increases it burns up everything in front of you? It burns up your family, your friends, your very sense of purpose in living. Or do you find a way to control it better and create a full life for yourself in spite of the pain you feel?

At some point in their travels through medical assessments, most of my patients have been told by a physician to "live" with their pain. Although I believe my colleagues are sincerely trying to be helpful, telling a patient to "live" with their pain tells me that the physician has never experienced it. In all my years of practice in the field of chronic pain, I have never told a patient to live with their chronic pain. That makes no sense to me. Why would anyone want to live with it? It's nothing but misery. Instead, I tell them that I might be able to show them how to live a better life in spite of the pain they feel. I am very honest. I tell them I might be able to help reduce their pain a bit, but I cannot make it go away. The proof is obvious. If I could make it go away, I would have done it for myself a long time ago. I help them reduce the pain if possible and then learn to get on with their lives in spite of whatever pain is still present.

I developed a pain program that teaches people how to live a better life in spite of the pain they feel. There are many parts to this program, but one thing I teach in every program is an introduction to self-hypnosis. Why? When I first started dealing with chronic pain there was no help for me. There were no pain specialists and no pain programs available. I was not ready for surgery. I was on my own. All I could see in front of me was a life of pain and disability. I felt doomed to accomplish nothing except to suffer every day. I made a conscious decision that I was not going to let that happen to me. I was offered codeine. But it gave me terrible side effects. It made me vomit continuously, without stopping, for hours until I got it out of my system, so I avoided codeine like poison. In those days, doctors would not use anything stronger. I really was on my own.

I accidentally found my way into learning about hypnosis. I'm not a good hypnotic subject like some people are. In fact, I'm close to the worst you could find. But I saw hope in the skill so I worked hard to develop it. I saw a possibility of controlling my pain for the first time. Hypnosis is about moving from the outside world to inside yourself. Once I got it, I made it a part of my life and have done so for over 30 years. I use it every day to get some control of my pain. I use other skills that I teach in our pain program, but self-hypnosis is a very important skill for me. It works almost every time, reducing my pain by up to 30 percent. Some of my patients can actually decrease their pain close to 100 percent. I'm not that fortunate, but for me, 30 percent is great because I have never taken a medication that does a better job. There are no side effects. I have seen the effect last for several hours in some patients. For me, I can get a good hour of relief and then I just do it again. Once you learn how to do it from an expert, it's free.

I am not suggesting that by learning self-hypnosis your pain will disappear and you can throw out your medications. What I am saying is that it is a potentially powerful, under-utilized skill for managing chronic pain. I can also say that it's not dangerous. You can't get addicted to it, or die from overuse as can happen to vulnerable people taking opioids. There will be no need for future guidelines lowering the frequency or length of time that you use self-hypnosis.

Travel with me in this book as I explain the ins and outs of hypnosis. By learning self-hypnosis, you will develop the skill to move your mind from paying attention to the outside world to paying attention to inside yourself. Once there, by using specific techniques you can learn how to reduce your pain. You will tap into skills you never knew you had but that have always been there. Travel with me from the outside in.

Notes

1. The CDC recommendation to reduce the maximum opioid dosage to 90 milligrams equivalent

per day has been very controversial in medical circles. It wasn't that anyone doubted that opioids are dangerous and potentially deadly. The issue, they say, was the CDC's upper limit. The number 90 seemed to be pulled out of the air. It didn't recognize that some people might feel less pain with a higher dose.

1

My Story

I still remember what it felt like to be normal. The last time was 45 years ago. I was 16. Up until then I felt like I could do anything I wanted to—and I pretty much did. I boxed, did martial arts, and swam miles at a time. I was on the track and field, wrestling, and gymnastic teams. I specialized on the pommel horse. I weightlifted and actually had a six pack. Everything changed in the blink of an eye.

I was at a gymnastic practice and my buddies and I were taking a break from our training. We decided to play a quick game of soccer and I was the goalie. There was a shot on the net, I twisted to stop it, and bang, my right knee dislocated. It was right out of its socket and wedged into the side of my leg. I fell to the floor in agony. I cannot remember the pain but I do remember the terrible agony, the fear, and the absolute terror. That terror has never left me. In truth, the idea of a dislocation is the only thing that really frightens me to this day. It was not until I was taken into surgery and put under anaesthetic in order to reduce the dislocation that the pain stopped.

This was the beginning of my long and complicated medical history. I don't like telling this story because it reminds me of a lot of negative, painful things. But I'm sharing it with you now because I want you to know I know what pain is, from the inside out. The things I know about pain and suffering do not all come from textbooks. Some do, because I am a physician and assistant clinical professor of medicine. But the most important parts of my understanding of pain and suffering come from my experience with it. So I will take you down this dark path not only so you know I'm with you, but also for another reason. I descended into my version of hell but, as you will see, I found a way to come back and live a full and engaged life.

After disclocating my knee, I did my best to forget about what had happened and after six weeks I was back at it, doing gymnastics again and high jumping on the track and field team. Then it happened again, this time when I was climbing a ladder at a rustic cabin in the country. My knee dislocated while I was halfway up the ladder. I had to be carried down by some big guys, who lifted me into the back of a truck and drove me to the nearest hospital. Three hours later I was once again knocked out in order to put my knee back in place. Four months later, I had surgery to stabilize my now very damaged knee joint. The pain from the surgery was terrible, and it took me a long time to recover. In fact, I was never the same. My career as a competitive athlete was over.

Around this time, while I was bending over a bathtub at home, I felt a deep painful twinge in my back. I remember slowly going out into the family room, where my father, a grey-haired, bespectacled, quiet-spoken man was sitting and reading a history book like he always did. The room was quiet. I didn't say anything but I slowly lay down on the carpeted floor. I rested for bit, then got back up and went back to the bathtub. I didn't tell anyone what had happened—I didn't want to complain. My father was so involved in his book, he never really noticed me, which was fine, because I didn't want to talk about it.

Over the next few years, I suffered silently as my back pain got progressively worse. Then, as the years went by, and quite out of the blue, I dislocated my shoulders and the bones in my hands and feet and both hips. It hurt terribly, but I didn't complain to my friends and family. My rationale was that it wouldn't make any difference if they knew. In fact, no one really knew what was happening to me until I got married to my high school sweetheart, Gilda. By then, I was 22. She was the first person I told about the dislocations. One day, she got to see it happen. We were having a small party, and I was deep-frying artichokes. I had just lifted up a wok filled with boiling oil when my left knee dislocated. The pan went flying and so did the oil.

Luckily no one was burned. I was writhing with pain on the floor while someone called an ambulance. Once again, I was taken to the hospital, knocked out, and my knee was put back in. Just before this dislocation, I was scheduled to have a revision surgery to my right knee because the original surgery had left me with a lot of pain. When I called the surgeon, a well-known author on the subject of back pain, and told him that I had dislocated my other knee his reply was "Left knee, right knee, I don't care." Well, I did. I never let that surgeon touch me.

By then I had a serious problem. Although I was only 24, my right knee had already deteriorated, and now my left knee was damaged too. I had to decide what to do. I met a new surgeon, who made a reasonable plan and did a Hauser procedure on my left knee. Although the procedure is not done anymore, it has worked for me all these years. The Hauser is referred to as a distal realignment procedure—in other words, the pull on the kneecap is being realigned to stop dislocations. I have never had problems with that knee and I will always be grateful to him.

Not long after, my father started having trouble with chest pain. He could not walk up our driveway without being short of breath. My dad was a pharmacist who was also a black belt in karate long before it became popular. Later in his career he left pharmacy and got his degree in education. After that he got a job teaching tough kids remedial classes in science and mathematics. He was a very gentle man and I always felt that we were close.

Unfortunately, he required bypass heart surgery, and the surgery changed him. We now know that the surgery can cause strokes because the patient's blood is bypassed from their heart into a machine for a period of time. The machine puts the patient at risk for a stroke. Although the likelihood of this happening has greatly reduced over time, in the 1970s when my father had the surgery, the risk was high. Unfortunately, my father died shortly after the surgery due to complications.

Four days later, I had an appointment with a well-known rheumatologist. He diagnosed me with Ehler-Danlos Syndrome (EDS), which is a genetic connective tissue disorder. It affects collagen, a structural protein that fills in spaces in the body and makes up tissue that holds muscle to bone and holds joints together. It contributes to the physical strength of skin, joints, muscles, ligaments, blood vessels, and visceral organs. When the collagen is abnormal, it can't hold joints together properly and this can lead to multiple dislocations of joints. Have you ever seen a circus performer who can bend themselves into odd shapes and even fold themselves into a small luggage trunk? That's EDS. I remember telling the doctor, "This makes absolutely no difference to me right now. My father passed away four days ago. However, I'm sure it will become important later." I was right. It did become more important.

At 31, I was accepted into medical school. I managed reasonably well until my final undergraduate clerkship year. I was studying internal medicine, and I was part of a team transferring a very large patient when my back went out. This time was worse than ever before. Lying on the floor of the patient's hospital bedroom, I felt humiliated. I had to be taken out of the room on a gurney. I was off work for weeks because I could not stand up. My back and leg pain were now out of control, and I underwent two back surgeries. They did not help—they made my back pain worse.

By now, Gilda and I had three boys under the age of four. It looked like I would not be able to finish medical school, go to work, or take care of my family. I could not even take care of myself. I was referred to a surgeon; he was my last hope as I thought my life was over. In the surgeon's waiting room, I couldn't even tolerate sitting. When the nurse came out to call me into his office, I was lying across the chairs in agony. I knew a lot about back surgery as I had read all the papers the surgeon had written about the topic. He seemed impressed by my knowledge.

He performed some terribly painful invasive tests, and in the end he told me I required a fusion of my back from L4 to S1—the lower back. He would take bone from my hip and use it to fuse the vertebrae together so there would be no movement anymore in that part of my back. He would use screws to hold me together. I had hope.

Unfortunately, before I could have the surgery I got very sick. I had returned to work and was on call as an intern in the hospital. One day I had terrible right-sided neck pain, and I felt generally unwell. I got progressively sicker as the day went on. I remember I admitted a patient to the hospital in the emergency room and then I lay down on the bed beside him. The emergency doctor assessed me and thought I had hurt my neck. He gave me a soft collar to wear and told me to come back if things got worse.

I went home after my shift, feeling very unwell. The next day was the second birthday of my second son, Daniel. Lots of family and friends were coming over. I went to bed hoping I would feel better the next day. I never made it to the party. I woke up in the middle of the night, feeling like a knife was being stuck and twisted into the right side of my neck. In agony, I told Gilda I had to go to the hospital. With three little boys at home, she could not go with me. I have no idea how I did it, but I drove myself to the hospital. I did not leave for over a month.

As I came into the emergency room, I still had searing pain in the right side of my neck, radiating into my right arm. Staff did not want to call the on-call neurologist because it was the middle of the night. They gave me codeine and I started vomiting. I spent hours writhing and vomiting in the emergency room until the neurologist arrived. After she assessed me, she told me I might have a brain stem tumour. The brain stem is that part of the brain that keeps us alive. It is responsible for keeping us breathing, maintaining our heart rate and blood pressure, and maintaining our temperature. A tumour in that part of the brain is fatal and the death is terrible.

I then had test after test. The neurologist also started to give me morphine, which settled the pain, but I continued to vomit. I had a lumbar puncture with a needle put in my spine to draw out fluid for testing. By this point my neck pain was even worse, and all the muscles on the right side of my neck started to atrophy, shrinking away along with my right shoulder; specifically affected were my deltoid muscle, trapezius, and other muscles of the rotator cuff. I was unable to lift my arm. My face slowly became paralyzed. I couldn't close my eyes. I couldn't swallow. I had trouble breathing. I could barely talk. A burning pain slowly covered my entire body in a weird patchy distribution.

After I'd spent a restless night, thinking about dying horribly, the neurology resident called to tell me that the test seemed to indicate I had a brain tumour. He hung up and left me with images of dying. I was worried about my family. What would they do for money? I had no insurance at that time. Then the chief of neurology called. In a staccato British accent, without a hint of feeling, he told me the resident was wrong; I did not have a brain tumour after all. I had Guillain-Barré Syndrome (GBS) and a weird form of it. I was diagnosed with a Miller Fischer form of GBS and a brachial neuritis. This meant I was in big trouble but at least it was not a brain stem tumour.

Guillain-Barré Syndrome is a nerve disease. Most nerves in the body have a covering called myelin. Without myelin, nerves do not transmit signals properly. In Guillain-Barré Syndrome, the myelin sheath of the nerves is stripped off because the patient's immune system attacks the nerves. Antibodies, which normally protect us from germs, attack the nerve cells and strip off the myelin. This condition is called an autoimmune disease. As a result, the nerves do not transmit signals properly, leading to what is called a flaccid paralysis. In a flaccid paralysis, it is as if the nerves to an area have been cut. If this happens in an arm or leg, the muscles lose all tone and the limb won't move. It can also happen to the muscles of the face, which is what happened with me.

The other diagnosis, brachial neuritis, is thought to be a massive inflammatory response that can be triggered by trauma, heredity, or unknown causes. It causes the nerves on the side of your neck to demyelinate, leaving the shoulder, arm, and neck weak and in terrible pain.

I had pain in my right, dominant arm from the neuritis, but I also had patches of burning pain all over my body from the GBS. It felt like someone had poured boiling water on me. Yet when I told the doctors and nurses I was in terrible pain, they thought it odd, and I felt they never really understood. At the time (the early 1990s), doctors didn't really consider how painful the disease can be. Now they do. The neurologist assigned to my case wasn't very sympathetic. When Gilda got to the hospital, she asked him if I was going to die. The neurologist shrugged his shoulders: "I don't know" was all he could think to say. My life was now in his hands. When you think about it, it's amazing that I survived. (What is funny is he is now in the same building that I work in. Every time I see him I want to hit him, but I control myself.)

Fortunately, not all the doctors were like him. I was hooked up with a haematologist because of the type of treatment I needed. Later, he became the dean of a major medical school. He was a wonderful man who, during my treatment, came in to see me on the weekends. I started a treatment called plasmapharesis. In the procedure, my blood was removed and put in a centrifuge, which spun it around so that the blood split into two parts, the cell component and the liquid component called plasma. The plasma was discarded, and I was offered the choice of fresh frozen plasma or saline, which is really salt water. I chose saline because I was worried about getting hepatitis from the plasma. My concerns were well founded. Everyone I knew with GBS at that time who had chosen fresh frozen plasma developed hepatitis. The only problem with saline was that it does not have all the components of plasma, so the treatments left me tired and exhausted. I was lucky however; the treatment helped. The muscle weakness started to reverse except in my right arm where I had the brachial neuritis. After a month of treatment, I was strong enough to leave the hospital.

When I was discharged, I was far from normal. I could not use my right arm, and it had to be wrapped up against my body, or the pain was out of control. I had burning over most of my body in a patchy distribution. I was weak. My eyes dried up and my mouth was constantly dry. I had to use eye drops all day and chew gum so my mouth was moist enough so I could still talk. The neurologist told me that it would take three years for my arm to recover but any damage that remained after that would be permanent. I was lucky. I can now use my right arm but I have very subtle damage left from the attack. I still have burning all over and dry eyes and mouth although not as intense as it once was. I was told that GBS can be a terrible disease but you have only one attack and you recover from it. I was past the worse, or so I thought.

A year almost to the day of my first attack, I had another attack after I caught a cold. My face and mouth became numb and I became terribly weak. I was sick again. It turned out I have a rare form of chronic Guillain-Barré syndrome, the kind that can come back, again and again. As a result I have to take strong doses of immunosuppressants. These medicines suppress my immune system so that it stops attacking my nerves. One of the medicines I take is a steroid, which is an old, very powerful immunosuppressant. The only problem is that steroids have tons of side effects—describing them could fill books. You have to be very careful with these types of medicines.

I have had multiple attacks of GBS. Some have been quite terrible. In my mid-40s, I stopped medication after a doctor told me my problems were all in my head. I didn't like taking the medications and hoped he was right, but three months later, I had the sudden onset of terrible searing pain in my right leg. Once again, I was writhing on the floor. It felt like someone was tearing the nerve out of my leg. Within minutes I could not stand up. My right leg was completely paralyzed. The pain was terrible. I could not sit and I thrashed for hours before the searing pain settled enough that I could even talk. Then came the rounds of doctors once again. I had tests and more tests, all of which told me what I knew already. The disease had stripped the nerve in my leg and it was paralyzed. The nerve had stripped the L5 nerve root of my right leg. The attack affected more than my leg. It also affected my hip so I could not hold my pelvis up.

The worst day of my life was when an occupational therapist came to my house to help me with mobility. She measured me for a walker. Then she started to measure me for a wheelchair. I was terrified—I was just 48 years old. I didn't let her finish this assessment. I felt that if I got a wheelchair I would never get out of it. I asked her nicely to leave. I was then put on high doses of my immunosuppressant, prednisone. The disease started to reverse.

What a mess. But don't forget, my back has always been a problem. When I'd had back surgery at age 35, I was sick, so I was considered high risk. Luckily for me, the surgeon believed in his own skills enough that he thought he could help me. Before the surgery he came into my room and said repeatedly, "You will not get sick," as though through his strength of will, I would be fine. I was desperate. On the day of the surgery, I told the surgeon, "If you can't help me, please don't wake me up." He did wake me up, and the surgery made a huge difference. My leg pain was almost gone and my back felt stronger, more stable. I did have a relapse of GBS right after the surgery, but I managed. The back pain has never gone away, but that surgery brought it down to a level where I could live life. I could even run after my children when they were little.

When I had my fusion, the surgeon said it would last 15 years. At the time it seemed like forever. He was close. It lasted 17 years before I needed another fusion. I am now fused from L3-S1. That's four levels. If I require one more fusion, they will have to fuse me from thoracic T10 down to S1. That's eight levels. I will have a lot of trouble moving so I've avoided this like poison.

Now, at age 62, I still have the sensation of a weird burning all over my face, hands, and feet. My hands ache all the time and it's very hard for me to hold a pen for any length of time because of the multiple dislocations of my thumb. I've had six hand surgeries to try to stabilize things. I have developed a problem with my right eye called an epi-retinal membrane. Scar tissue inside the eye is pulling on the retina, distorting my vision. To correct it could require a very risky eye surgery.

I've had plenty of surgeries over the last few years. I've had many painful attacks of the paralyzing GBS, including one horrible one while writing this book, and I'm bound to have more. But in spite of it, I still do my best to have what I feel is a very full life. I still work full-time—well, 95 percent of the time. There is the odd day when I have difficulty, but I make those as rare as possible. Why do I push myself to work? I get a lot from my patients. In truth, by hearing their stories, I forget about mine. If I can help someone, it makes my own misery worthwhile. Some people ask me how I handle patients' complaints when their problems are trivial compared to mine. I don't think about it that way. Their problems are theirs. If having a hangnail is destroying their lives, then that is what they need help with. It makes no difference how bad their physical problem is.

When I'm not working, I'm always busy. It's the way I cope. I rarely stop. If I stop, I start thinking about what's hurting and then it just hurts more. I have a shop and a studio where I build boats and paint. I built my first boat when I was 23, right after my second knee surgery. I had been a keen canoeist and used to race canoes but now I couldn't kneel in a canoe because of the pin in the middle of my kneecap. It was too painful to put pressure on it. So I decided to build a sailboat. Eleven years later, I was hospitalized with GBS. This time, not only could I not canoe, but I couldn't do anything very physical with my three little boys. I couldn't play hockey with them. I couldn't even throw a ball. It was then that I decided to build a boat, and although I was someone who always worked with a self-imposed deadline I set no timeline for its completion. My sons could come out and help me. The youngest was just about two years old so I had to make special tools for him. That's when the boat building started, and since then we've built 10 canoes, sailboats, and kayaks, including several canoes with clear bottoms that allow you to see the water below as you paddle. We use them every summer and watch the fish swimming under the canoe as we paddle. One of the canoes with a clear bottom hangs in the front hall of our home the rest of the year. I still canoe. I can still do things in a canoe that most people can't. I just can't do it for very long sometimes. But I can do it long enough and I can go canoeing with Gilda and that's all I need. We canoe for hours at a time talking and trying to sneak up on loons.

I cope with my pain by doing. After every surgery or relapse, I launch a project. I've had 12 episodes and that's why I have at least 12 projects on the go. I'm building three different boats—a trimaran, a sloop-rigged sailboat, and a cedar strip canoe. One project is an elastic-band Gatling gun. I'm building a music box and a clock. I've started making a very elaborate dragon puzzle and a complex whirligig. I'm also building a classical guitar and a beautiful coffee table with a lift top and four drawers. I've built several take-down recurve bows and one of them has a sight system that I invented. I'm building a primitive native bow made from osage orangewood backed by animal tendon and hide glue. I'm building a 10-inch telescope, and if this goes well, I'll attempt a 12-inch telescope. For me, it never stops. There is always something new to try.

At my most sick or impaired, I start to think about a new building project and when I'm well enough, I start it. As I tell people, if I live long enough, I'll finish every project!

By creating positive goals when I'm at my worst, I cope with the bad cards I have been dealt.

I've been painting since before I could write. I use all types of media and always find something new to try. Most recently I started painting in encaustic, a very ancient art form that involves painting with wax. The Egyptians covered their mummies in encaustic art. There is always something new to discover that makes life interesting in spite of not feeling very well.

I love magic. My uncle Jack showed me an amazing magic "effect" (magicians don't say tricks—dogs do tricks, magicians do magic) when I was about nine years old. From that day on I wanted to know how to do magic. Now I can do some pretty complicated magic. I taught my sons, and they used to go into hospitals and do magic shows for the children there. If ever there was a distraction from feeling lousy, magic is it.

Last, I cook and I bake. In fact, my wife and I are working on a cookbook together. She is an amazing cook in spite of the fact that when we got married she couldn't cook at all. I taught her and she took it from there. When I'm cooking, I can forget about how I feel and I get the added pleasure of watching someone else enjoy what I've made. It has nothing to do with being unwell. All the things I do help me feel "normal."

My life might have been very different if none of this had occurred. Perhaps I would have been a surgeon and maybe I would still be boxing. Who knows? In spite of everything,

I am still able to contribute to the lives of people, teach medical students something about pain, and contribute to the medical literature. I build beautiful boats, play a mean guitar, and create some wonderful paintings. Not bad for such a messed-up guy.

2

One Goal at a Time

At the worst point of my life, when I was paralyzed in hospital, deep in pain, I truly believed that the only way I was going to recover was by the strength of my own will, plus a bit of luck and some clever, understanding physicians. I realized there were certain things I could not control, like the disease I had and how it would proceed. It could affect my breathing and if it did I would land up on a respirator. I could not control how much permanent damage the disease would cause. I could not control my response to any treatment provided. If I could not control it, I did not think about it. I decided I needed clear and positive goals to think about. I needed goals that had nothing to do with where I was and nothing to do with being sick. Having goals would give me some control.

First I decided I was going to finish medical school. Given where I was, it seemed a bit ridiculous. There was a good chance that even if I survived, I would be paralyzed. So that wasn't necessarily a realistic goal. However, it was a long-term plan. A goal is what you can do right now. It might be a small step toward a bigger goal or, in my case, long-term plan. Although I could not stand independently, I decided to make my bed. If I could make my bed, I knew I would survive and get out of the hospital. Maybe I would even be able to walk by myself. If I could walk again, maybe I could go back to work. If this happened, I would be an intern in medical school again.

The nurses put me in a wheelchair, and I slowly worked my way around the bed by myself. It took me about two hours but I did make the bed. I even included hospital corners. It doesn't seem like much now but given how sick and weak I was, it was a miracle. This was one of the biggest accomplishments of my life, and still is. I have never forgotten it and now I start my day with that same goal. I start my day by making my bed. I know that if I make my bed, everything else I do that day is a bonus. If I can't make the bed, it means I'm very sick and in serious trouble. There have been some days when I haven't made the bed, but those days are few and far between. Making the bed reminds me of where I was and how far I've come. When you are injured or become sick, start thinking of goals that are about living life, not about being sick.

I started by making the bed. Then I got out of the hospital. Then I was able to feed myself, and then I was able to walk. Eventually I went back to work as a doctor. It was difficult for me. When I started back at work, my right arm was paralyzed and had to be tied tightly against my body or the pain was out of control. I used an electronic board to write my notes with my left hand. Fortunately, I'm comfortably ambidextrous. Perfecting the hospital corner had been a start, but I had to contend with a much deeper issue. What was I going to do with my life? Before I got sick, I was a very physical person. In those days, I thought I was going to be a competitive athlete and a surgeon. Suddenly I could do very little by comparison. I was a patient, with a rare and bizarre disease. I suddenly felt like my life had no meaning. Once I started to be able to think clearly again, I realized I had to find new meaning in my life. Although I had no idea how impaired I was going to be, that uncertainty didn't make a difference. I had to find some kind of meaning in my life regardless of my impairment or the disease would win, it would destroy my life—and drag down everyone I cared about with me.

Even while I was in the hospital, I thought there had to be some way to make use of what was happening to me. I was lucky that I was in medicine. There are so many opportunities in the profession. I just had to find something that fit my new physical abilities and limitations. I had always wanted to be a surgeon and in fact had been accepted into a program for otolaryngology (ears, nose, and throat, commonly referred to as ENT). This opportunity was gone. I could not even sit up independently at this time. I thought about primary care. At first it seemed that I could manage it. However, when I went back to work, starting in primary care, the physical demands were too much for me. Still, I decided that no matter how sick I was or how limited I was I was going to become a practising physician. Rather than thinking about myself, I wanted to be a practising doctor who helped other people. I thought this way I could still contribute no matter how sick I was.

Given my condition, psychiatry seemed to be the best bet. After all, I had my Master's Degree in Social Work and I could build on those skills in psychiatry. It all seemed to make sense. I was accepted into the residency. In my third year, I did part of my psychiatric training in New Zealand. Gilda and our three small sons joined me there. We were there for four months. However, the flight back home was 23 hours, and by the time we touched down I was starting to relapse from my immunologic disease. It took months to recover. It always does. At the time, Gilda was working as a physiotherapist at the only chronic pain program in the Hamilton-Wentworth Niagara region of Ontario. While I was recovering from this latest attack, Gilda and her colleagues came up with a plan. They decided I should do a rotation at their program. I met with the director of the program, a well-known, somewhat eccentric psychiatrist. At our first meeting, he said, "Come and do what you can." That was unheard of in a residency program. Usually supervisors are more like friendly vampires. They do their best to suck out as much work from you as possible, but they do it nicely. Yet here was a supervisor who told me to do what I can. At that time my capacity wasn't much. Yet it turned out to be enough. I discovered that having major problems myself was a big asset with most pain patients. I really do understand what they're going through.

Before I finished my residency, I was invited to become the director of the outpatient pain program. It was in danger of being closed down, and I was given the job of reviving it. I worked there for five years and then launched my own pain program. Initially, we partnered with a local hospital. Over time I decided to move away from hospital politics and started my own program. At first it was called the East End Pain Program. The name was then changed to the Ennis Centre for Pain Management. Now, 18 years later I can honestly say that I have never turned a patient away due to lack of money. If patients have no money, I subsidize them. However, these patients have a single payment. They have to buy me a cup of coffee. That's it.

Our pain program is not about pain reduction. I wish I could do that—I would be feeling a lot better than I do if I could. But I can't. I do show some techniques like acupressure and self-hypnosis that can help reduce pain but that is not the main point of the program. The purpose of the program is to get people back into life. The idea is to learn to live life *in spite* of the pain you have, not learn to *live with* your pain. When people get sick or have a traumatic injury, their lives change. Suddenly they are not working. Other people expect very little from them. They develop a "disabled lifestyle." They get up late in the morning because no one is waiting for them. No one cares. They might meet a friend for a coffee. They might lie down in the afternoon and watch some television. They become progressively weaker and less important in the world. Soon, everyone they know expects nothing from them and friends fall away, leaving the patient more isolated and alone. The person's life is now meaningless, without purpose.

My program is all about function and the search for meaning. It is about how to re-engage in living again so the patient's life does matter and has a sense of purpose. It is about being able to move in the world again and not let pain run a person's life. The program has a lot to do with changing how a person thinks about themselves and about their pain. As an old volunteer of mine always says, "When I came into the program, pain was running my life. Now, I run my life." I think that says it all.

In our pain program, we formalize the whole business of goal setting. It is central to what we do. We show patients how to set basic, small, do-able goals that are SMART.

S *means specific.* Your goal must be carefully crafted and be clear and specific as to what you plan to do. "I want to be a millionaire" is not a goal. It is a wish. "I will save ten dollars every week" is a goal.

M *stands for measureable.* The goal must be measured so you can tell if you are attaining it. "I will exercise" is not measureable. "I will exercise for 20 minutes three days a week" is measureable.

A *stands for achievable.* Do not set goals you cannot reach. A goal for me of running for one kilometre is simply not achievable. My back is fused and my knees are badly damaged. "I will walk a quarter of a kilometre three times a week" is achievable in my current state. If I start with this goal, perhaps I can increase the distance I walk or the frequency of walking with time.

R *is for relevant.* No point is choosing a goal that has no meaning for you. "I will grow my hair to my shoulders" is not a meaningful goal for me now although it was when I was 17 and I did accomplish it ... then.

T *is for time-bound.* To keep a goal relevant it needs to have a boundary of time around it to keep you moving forward. "I will exercise in a year" is not a meaningful goal. "I will exercise three times per week, for 15 minutes each time, starting tomorrow" is time-bound.

Patients are instructed to write goals every day and evaluate them. They have to ask themselves a couple of questions: What helped to achieve their goals? What got in the way? How well did they do? Does the goal need to be rewritten? If so, they need to make the necessary adjustments and start over. I've been doing this for close to 30 years now and it moves me forward. The literature is very clear. Simply by writing down a goal, a patient is likely to show some improvement. Setting goals can be very powerful.

We also provide information, lots of information. The more a person understands what is happening to them, the better they will cope. It helps patients make reasonable decisions. We have many sessions, including sessions about chronic pain medications, fitness, productivity, sexuality, nutrition, sleep, and the use of laughter in coping. We're happy to field any question. I have never had a patient who has asked a foolish question. If I don't know the answer to their question, I will find the answer. Knowledge is a powerful tool in coping with chronic pain.

We also have very specific fitness sessions. This is not quite the same as physiotherapy. Physiotherapy will not help chronic pain as much as patients would like. It is much more useful for acute injuries. Going to the gym without knowing what you are doing is also not helpful. In fact, it can be potentially dangerous. We show people a very specific, safe program of exercise that they can do on their own. Many patients carry on with the program after we finish the group and they become stronger and are able to manage their pain better.

We do tai chi. People learn the Chen style, consisting of 37 movements. It helps people become less fearful of moving, is a very safe form of exercise, and is a lot of fun. Although I have run the program for 20 years, I did not learn the 37 moves until quite recently. This was when my wife Gilda was diagnosed with breast cancer and had to have chemotherapy. I decided that I had to come up with ways for us to do enjoyable things together so that her months of chemo would not turn into a complete misery. My wife had chemo every other Friday, so every other Friday in between we went to tai chi. My instructor and friend, Mike, gave his time and expertise to teach us this wonderful program of exercise. We practise almost every night. Recently, on New Year's Day, we showed all our children the 37 moves. I think they were impressed. I know I was. Now we both know these moves and have moved on to tai chi using fans. After that, swords!

Our program has an aquatherapy component. Patients exercise in a pool under the supervision of a pool therapist. It helps people become stronger and, again, less fearful of movement.

We teach multiple modalities that people can use to help control their pain. These include a wide array of relaxation strategies. They begin by learning relaxation in the most ideal condition possible: sitting in a comfortable chair in a quiet room. However, by the end of the program, they have learned to do relaxation in order to control their pain while standing in a busy place. Otherwise the skill is not very useful in day-to-day life. We don't use tapes to teach relaxation. I've seen hundreds of patients who've been given relaxation tapes by a therapist. The only thing these tapes might do is make the person who recorded the tape a bit more wealthy. Patients who use these tapes do not learn a useful, transportable skill. They go home and listen to the tape. They are not in the outside world. The purpose of learning this skill is to increase mobility, not decrease it. Unless a clinician is helping a patient use the relaxation tape to learn the skill so that they can do it independently in the real world, it is not very helpful. I also teach acupressure so people have a way to control pain.

Finally, I introduce my groups to self-hypnosis. Some of these patients go on to our 10-week hypnotherapy program. The first five sessions of the hypnotherapy program focus on learning the skills of self-hypnosis. By session five of the hypnotherapy program , I start to teach hypnosis for pain control, and by session 10, the vast majority of patients can control their pain better than when we began. For many, this is the first time they have felt relief without side effects. We'll describe the techniques of self-hypnosis for pain control later in this book.

As you can see, our pain program has multiple components. For effective pain control, you need all parts of our multi-dimensional pain program. No single tool will do it all. This is because chronic pain is a complex problem involving brain and body. It's very different from acute pain, as we shall see in the next chapter.

3

What You Need to Know About Chronic Pain

It still surprises me that even though nearly 30 per-cent of Canadians live with chronic pain, the majority of physicians are not well trained in this important field. When I was in medical school, we did not have a single lecture on pain. Not one. It's odd because chronic pain is so common and destructive. Pain is an important human issue. In fact, in 1999, the U.S. Veterans Health Administration put forward the concept that pain should be treated as the fifth vital sign after blood pressure, temperature, pulse rate, and respiratory rate.

That was more than 15 years ago, and yet still today, many physicians do not know very much about pain. That is why you, as a patient, need to understand the fundamentals of chronic pain. The more you know, the better you will be able to handle your own problems and help your physicians think more about your problems.

Why do we feel pain? It's unpleasant. What's the point? In fact, the physiology of pain was probably in place when the first organism showed itself on earth. The ability to feel pain is in all animal life. There is even some evidence that plants respond to what they perceive as painful stimuli. They will move away from loud noises. Single-cell organisms will swim away from bright lights. All animals feel pain. It's there for a purpose. In fact, without it, we could not survive. We have examples from diseases in which pain is not felt anymore. The most concerning disease is congenital insensitivity to pain. The affected person does not feel pain and as a result has rotting teeth, multiple unfelt fractures, untreated infection, and the possibility of potentially fatal untreated disease. These patients do not live full lives. It is also possible to have a later onset of being unable to feel pain in a disease called Charcot joints or neuropathic joints. The causes could be spinal injury, diabetes, or syphilis. The result is that the nerves going to joints are damaged and do not transmit the sensation of pain. In such a condition, the person does not adjust their position like other people do all day, resulting in the joints slowly dissolving over time. Fortunately, the disease is not seen much anymore but it nicely illustrates the point that you must be able to feel pain in order to survive.

We all feel pain, and yet it's hard to define. The International Association for the Study of Pain (IASP) described pain this way: "An unpleasant sensory and emotional experience associated with actual or potential tissue damage, or described in terms of such damage." It's not surprising that when you get a bunch of physicians together they come up with a definition that is difficult to decipher. What this definition means is that pain is not just the physical "hurting" from an injury or disease. Pain also has an *emotional* component. Think about it. When you have pain, don't you feel upset, depressed, or angry? Only the odd individual likes it. The emotional aspect of pain is hardwired. It's a physical and emotional sensation.

Now that you know what pain is, it is important to know that there are three types of pain: acute pain, cancer pain, and chronic pain. They are all different. Acute pain is the pain you feel after an acute trauma like breaking your leg. That hurts immediately. Acute pain is expected to go away after a while, when the injury heals.

Cancer pain comes from a cancerous growth invading some part of the body and causing pain because of it. Sometimes cancer pain can be the result of a paraneoplastic syndrome—a secondary disease caused by the cancer itself. Cancer can also cause pain because of the general debility of the patient, the terrible immobility caused by the disease.

What about chronic pain? What is it? I'll give you an example of what it is not. I consulted with a colleague of mine a number of years ago because of problems with my hips. He's a very bright fellow. He was well aware of my complex history, and in an effort to be empathic he said, "I had chronic pain once." Like a good psychiatrist, I asked for clarification and he repeated his statement. I gently pointed out to him that he was not quite accurate. If he had the pain only once, it means that his pain was now gone. If his pain was gone now, it was not chronic. I'm not sure he got the point. The point is chronic pain is not pain lasting longer than three or six months as physicians are taught. It is pain that will never go away. Never, ever go away. That's quite different than acute pain, which has a beginning and an end. Cancer pain and chronic pain share the likelihood that both of these pains will not go away. Unfortunately, the pain of cancer can be associated with the end of life; if the cancer can be reversed, the pain typically goes away or reduces because the invading tumour has reduced or disappeared. Cancer pain is treated very differently than chronic pain. The focus of cancer pain treatment is to eradicate the cancer if possible and decrease the pain as best as possible so that a person is as comfortable as possible. Function is not as concerning an issue. Medications are used even if they might negatively affect function. The focus is on the pain.

Chronic pain treatment is different—we try not to use medications that impede function. The pain is not indicative of a life-ending disease. Our goals are twofold, to decrease pain and to increase function with an expectation of continued life.

In order to understand chronic pain, it is very important to understand the neurophysiology of acute pain. The neuroanatomical pathways of pain used to be thought of in a very straightforward manner. You hurt something and the signal goes to your brain. The brain interprets the signal as pain and now you feel it. In fact, the physiology of pain is much more complicated. Imagine you hit your finger with a hammer. Receptors in your finger called nociceptors turn on and send the pain signal from the finger, down the arm to the spine. Then the signal travels up the spine to a part of the brain called the thalmus, deep in the cortex of the brain, which then relays that information to the pain matrix. The pain matrix is made up of a very specific part of the brain called the sensory cortex where pain is felt and localized but it also includes the limbic system, which is the emotional part of the brain. That is why the physical sensation of pain is associated with negative emotional changes.

The stimulation of negative emotions caused by pain is meant to be a learning pathway. Think about something painful that happened to you. Do you actually remember the physical pain? Probably not. If we remembered that kind of pain, no one would have more than one child. What we remember is the negative emotional part of pain. Generally, birth pain is a positive pain, so we have families with more than one child. The pain does not have a terrible negative association in memory. But I bet you won't stick your hand in a fire if you've been burnt before. You remember the fear, terror, and perhaps anger of the trauma. You have an emotional response to the pain and you have thoughts about what it means, which typically leads to an action.

When the pain signal gets to the brain, the spine and the brain try their best to control pain, to reduce it if possible. How? First, all humans have naturally occurring opioids called endogenous opioids that are secreted after trauma or even under stress. They work just like morphine and are designed to reduce pain. In addition, complex signals descend from the brain after a painful event to try to control the pain. Multiple sites in the brain are involved with the two most important areas, called the periaqueductal grey (PAG) and the raphe nucleus (RN).

There is one more phenomenon worth knowing about. It is called the gating or gate control theory and was elucidated by Ronald Melzak, a Canadian psychologist, and Patrick David Wall, a British neuroscientist, in the 1960s. The theory continues to be influential in the field of pain management. It is a complex theory but here it is in its simplest form: there is a pain control mechanism in the spinal cord that can be stimulated by touch, vibration, or pressure. These stimuli "close the gate" on pain. They block it. Pain is reduced. This means nonpainful stimulation can reduce pain. The simplest example of gating is rubbing your finger after you hit it with a hammer. Why do you rub the area? It reduces pain.

What happens with chronic pain? This becomes a bit more involved than acute pain. Let's start at the beginning, although in this case the beginning is a bit different. The nociceptors in your finger turn on, just as they do after you hit your finger with a hammer, but other receptors get activitated too. These are wide dynamic range receptors, and they spread the pain from where it began.

Now let's head to the spine. In acute pain, the pain signal goes up the spine, but in chronic pain the spine becomes excitable because of the constant pain signals travelling up it. Eventually the spine develops a lower threshold for firing off pain signals.

Now let's go to the brain. A few things are happening here. First, the pain signals do not just go to the pain matrix as they do in acute pain. The signals go to a few other spots in the brain and get spread around a bit. So now multiple areas of the brain are involved in processing the pain signals. It is unclear exactly what this means but what it does tell us is that there have been changes in the brain as a result of a chronic pain signal. Some of the phenomena I've just described are part of a new area of research called neuroplasticity. We used to think that when you became an adult, the brain was, in effect, frozen—it did not and could not change. Now we know that is not true. The brain has plasticity—it can change even in adulthood. In chronic pain, this neuroplasticity sets up memories of pain that are very hard to get rid of.

Other changes occur in the brain. We now know that certain areas of the brain actually shrink in the face of chronic pain, and the longer the pain is present, the more the brain shrinks. There is also evidence that different parts of the brain start talking to each other. The conversation between parts of the brain in chronic pain is different than it is in acute pain. All these changes can have an impact on the sensory, emotional, and modulatory circuits of the brain. Overall, the brain appears to be widely affected by chronic pain. However, I like to think that if the brain can change in a negative direction then it should be able to change in a positive direction too. I should be able to teach myself how to handle my pain better, and if I do that then the plasticity of my brain will allow these positive changes to become more permanent.

No wonder people feel so miserable. Clearly, chronic pain is a different entity than acute pain. But that's not all. If you have chronic pain, you'll find that your loved ones and friends treat you very differently than they would if you broke a leg. Say you fell off your bike and fractured your leg. You go to the hospital and the attending doctor has a pretty good idea of what is wrong from the get-go and feels confident she can help. Imaging is done and, voilà, a fracture is seen. Let's assume it's an uncomplicated fracture. A cast is applied and you're sent home with a note from the doctor for your boss that you need time off work.

At home, you lie down. Everyone agrees you should lie down. After all, you're in pain. Family and friends swarm around to help. Someone is bound to make chicken soup. You're not expected to help clean up. You might even get a sympathetic call from work, plus some flowers. You go for your follow-up to the doctor. She takes an X-ray again and tells you the bone is healing well and the cast will come off pretty soon.

You have an injury but you feel cared for. Work is paying you and everyone seems so supportive. Off comes the cast and you go for physiotherapy to strengthen your weak leg. After a few weeks, you're almost all better. You go back to work and over time everything is back to normal.

Sounds great, doesn't it? It might even be worth having a fracture to get all that support and attention. Now let's look at chronic pain. Say you had a very bad back injury. You are progressively more impaired until you have surgery. You end up with six back surgeries. Now your back hurts all the time. It has impaired your ability to work, and now you're getting long-term disability—66 percent of your salary—so you have a lot less money now. The telephone calls and flowers from work stopped coming a long time ago. Colleagues stopped dropping by because you can't do the things they like to do. You lie down almost all the time because of pain, and because you're not using your muscles you get weak. Now you have pain in other places too.

You don't help with chores, so your wife has to do everything. She's upset. Then the surgeon informs you that the surgery was successful and there's nothing more he can do. You turn to your family doctor to get painkillers, but you feel like your doctor is frustrated with your persistent calls and doesn't like prescribing the medicines.

In chronic pain, most systems break down. Work, family, friends, and medical systems falter. When we use the same methods of coping with acute pain for chronic pain, we are screwed. Acute pain is a system designed to make us stop, back off, rest, and seek help. Eventually you get better. We are designed to behave like that automatically regardless of the cause of the pain. That's why so many people behave like that with chronic pain. The problem is if you do that with chronic pain, it won't help. Your physical health will decline, and the pain will never stop, so you never stop seeking help. It rarely, if ever, works out.

It is clear that the world of chronic pain is very different than the acute pain world. Most people with chronic pain have lost their friends, are isolated, do very little, and feel useless and guilty about not contributing to their family's well-being. They are made poorer by their physical problems, and most of the time none of it was their fault.

As a pain specialist, I do use medicines to try to help reduce a person's chronic pain as part of an overall strategy to get out of the rut of chronic pain and get their lives back. The primary goal is to increase their function. But as you will see in the next chapter, I prescribe pain medications with great caution—medicines are not the final answer to the problem.

4

The Problem
With Pills

When we have pain, we go to the doctor, and we assume that they will come up with a plan to help us. Nine times out of ten, that means using medications. That's what the public thinks doctors do—prescribe medicines. In fact, for many people, if they do not get a medicine from their doctor, they feel undertreated, even cheated somehow.

Unfortunately, in chronic pain, it's rare to find a medicine that actually makes the pain go away. I have a host of medicines at my disposal, and yet for the over 20 years I have been in the field of chronic pain, I have had only one home run. That's right: one. This patient has an uncommon condition called burning mouth syndrome. In this syndrome, the patient's mouth burns as if it were full of scalding water. It can affect every aspect of the mouth, even the teeth. The only problem is, there is no obvious pathology causing the pain. I began treating her with gab-apentin, a drug that quiets down nerve transmission, and the pain went away. It went away completely and absolutely. It was an amazing home run, the only one I have ever had.

You would think we could do better. Millions and millions of dollars are spent every year trying to find that special medicine to take away the pain so many of us feel. A number of years ago, an Irish company began doing research on deep sea snails called cone snails. These little beasts eat their food alive because the venom they inject into their prey is about 10,000 times more potent than morphine. At the time, when studies were started on humans it was discovered that people hallucinate on this medication, called conotoxin. As the years have passed, the company did a lot of work and this venom, called ziconotide, is now available in rare cases. The problem is that it is given intrathecally, or into the spinal canal, and it can still make people hallucinate. Research is currently underway to try to find a way to make this medication available in a pill form with fewer side effects. Let's face it, if medications worked, there would be no need for the specialized programs I have developed to help people like me cope with the pain. Truth is, no one thing works for pain. A bit of this and a bit of that can make a big difference sometimes, and that's why I started doing hypnosis. It was not because medicines failed me. It was because medicines were not enough. Not only is it unlikely that medicines will take away your pain completely, but they typically come with consequences. They have side effects, and some are most unpleasant. If you are going to use medicines to help you with your pain, make sure that you understand everything you can about them.

There are way too many medicines to go through one by one in this book. Besides, it's easy to find out on the Internet about what medicines might do and their side effects. Instead I'm going to show you some clear examples of pitfalls with medicines, some of which you probably never knew existed. By the end you should be a much better informed patient.

What separates doctors from everybody else in our society is that we are permitted to prescribe medicines to people. This is an ancient art, dating back thousands of years to when the shaman of a tribe gave a patient the root or bark of a tree to cure an illness. The tradition of the shaman evolved over time but his skills are preserved in today's physicians. Early pharmaceuticals were based on what was found in nature—my pharmacist father had a pharmaceutical collection made up of bugs and roots and bark, all with medicinal characteristics. Over time we have been able to synthesize what nature has provided. Finally, we have branched out beyond nature and we synthesize our own medicines that are unique. What some medicines share is that, taken in sufficient quantity, they can be poisonous. As I tell all my new students: "You are now just like James Bond. As a doctor you are licensed to kill. Almost every medicine you prescribe is a potential poison. The trick is to give just enough that it is helpful and not so much that it is harmful." I try my best to scare them into respecting the use of medicines.

This is the basis of the pharmaceutical practice of medicine and it really has not changed very much from the time of the shaman. Just like the shaman, I can still kill a person with medicine.

There is a case that I tell all my patients. It has an important lesson about more not always being better. The patient, who was 23 years old, was referred to me to help her learn to cope better with the pain that she had from a very serious fracture of a leg. By the end of the program, she was coping much better. One year almost to the date from the last time I saw her, her primary care physician called me to tell me that this patient was dead. She died, by accident, because she took too much acetaminophen, one of the most common analgesics pain killers. She did not mean to do it. She just kept taking 15 to 20 pills of acetaminophen every day. The upper limit is 4 grams a day and she was taking up to 7 grams per day. This is not a prescription medication so she could buy as much as she wanted to. He told me that the medication had poisoned her so badly that she could not have a liver transplant in order to save her life. Her brain was already too damaged.

This is an example of pharmacokinetics at its worse. Pharmacokinetics focuses on the fate of a drug from the moment it is administered up to the point at which it is completely eliminated from the body. This examination includes where it goes in the body, how it is changed in the body, and how the body eliminates it. When you take a medication, the body works hard to get rid of it. One of the ways it does this is to make it soluble in water so it goes out in your urine. This action takes place in the liver, whose primary purpose is to keep our blood clean. One of its tricks is to attach certain molecules onto medications. It actually changes the molecular makeup of the medicine to make the drug more water soluble so it can be eliminated via the urine. In the case of acetaminophen, though, the new molecular makeup that the liver creates is extremely poisonous. That is why people can kill themselves by intention or by accident using acetaminophen.

The next thing to understand about a medication is how does it do what it is suppose to do. For example, how does aspirin reduce fever? How does the drug work? Physicians can learn how a medicine works at the molecular level. This is called pharmacodynamics. When physicians prescribe a medication, they should be very familiar with that medicine's pharmacokinetics and pharmacodynamics.

Medicines are a very big part of medical practice and they are everywhere in our culture. How do we know that they do what they are supposed to do and that they are safe to take? The answer is research. Research has become very sophisticated. Medicines go through many levels of research for many years before they are released by a company for human consumption. It costs hundreds of millions of dollars to bring a medicine to market.

It is very important for me as a doctor to understand the research about the medicines I use for patients. It is equally important for me as a patient to have some idea about the research related to the medicines I take so that I know what to expect and how to take care of myself in the best way possible.

In earlier days, researchers would give a medicine to a group of people and observe what happened. Did they get better or did they get worse? Did they get a few easy-to-handle side effects or terrible side effects? Sounds reasonable, doesn't it? Well, it's not. The problem is how do you know that the results you see are not because of something other than the medication used? What if it was simply due to the passage of time that it took to do your observation? What if it was due to changes in the seasons?

To answer this question, you need a control group. At its most basic, a control group is a group of people who do not get the intervention—like the medicine you're testing—while your other group gets it. You then compare the results of the two groups. If the group getting the medicine does better than the group that didn't, you might conclude that it was because of the medicine. This type of research is called a control trial.

Now if you really want to have a gold standard for a research trial, here's what you do: you select a group of people for the trial, then you select who gets the drug. All patients for both groups are selected *on a random basis*. And of course, you don't tell each person in the trial whether they're getting the drug or an inactive medication, the placebo. Also, you make sure the researchers do not know who is getting what. This is called "blinding." By doing this, you have reduced the likelihood that a patient gets a better result because they know the medication they are getting is the active one. Believe it or not, if the researcher knows who is getting what, this can also influence the outcome. It's called e-bias and there is a huge literature on this subject alone. This type of trial, where the patients and the researchers do not know who is getting the active medication, is called a double blind randomized control trial. This is the type of research you want to pay attention to and take seriously. You do not need to know the super complex aspects of this type of research but it is important to know the background if you want to know if the medicine you are taking has been researched using the gold standard. If you don't know this information, do not rush to take the medicine. Even if the medication has been researched in this way, you still have to ask your doctor three questions before you take the medicine.

What is the likelihood that this medicine will help me?

What is the likelihood that this medicine will harm me, and if it does harm me, how serious is the harm?

How good is the research?

Let's take these questions one by one.

Will It Help?

The question appears quite specific but it is not that simple. It depends on what the question is really asking. Is it "Does the medication reduce pain?" Or is it "Does it reduce pain so that function is improved?" My area in pain management focuses on coping and function. Function means being able to get up every day and do something that you enjoy and perhaps even makes you feel useful. To be truthful, if a treatment does not help to improve function, I am not very interested in it. A patient taking a medicine and telling me it reduces their pain, but they are lying in bed all day is not being helped very much, in my opinion. I have had colleagues criticize me about this stance. They have said, "Don't you think that reducing pain, whether a person does more or not, is our duty?" Well, I have an advantage over them; I'm a patient with some serious medical problems. I use these medicines. I hate them, but I use them. If you're going to use medicines that can cause serious problems like addiction, then you had better get a really good bang for your buck, and pain reduction without improved function is insufficient for me. Now remember, there is pretty good evidence for using a medicine like opioids for acute pain, such as pain from a fracture or a shrapnel injury in wartime. But for us, the real question is this: What is the evidence that it works for *chronic pain*, like back pain, the kind of pain that will never go away?

If we consider the question of whether a drug reduces pain, medicine has a statistical tool at the ready. It's called the numbers needed to treat or NNT. This is a measurement that refers to the number of people who must be treated by a specific intervention for one person to receive a certain effect. If I invented a new analgesic, and its number needed to treat was 1, it means every single person who uses it gets at least a 50 percent reduction in pain. A miracle! In the case of oxycodone (the medicine in Percocet), it turns out that 46 people have to be treated so that 10 of them feel 50 percent better. It has an NNT of 4.6. If you add acetaminophen to it, the result gets better. Only 27 people have to be treated so that 10 feel 50 percent better. Its NNT drops to 2.7. If you use an antiinflammatory (NSAID—nonsteroidal anti-inflammatory drug) like ibuprofen and add acetaminophen to it, the NNT is 1.6. Now that's impressive. In other words, 16 people have to be treated so that 10 feel 50 percent better. This suggests that in general NSAIDs are more effective than opioids. You just have to be careful about side effects.

But did you notice something? Even in the best-case scenario, some people don't get better, and the people that do get better do not necessarily feel no pain. They get 50 percent better.

Will It Hurt?
Then there is the issue of side effects. It is uncommon to find a medicine that does not cause side effects. Sometimes we don't know how serious some side effects are until

the medicine has been around for a while. The real issue is whether the side effects will do you harm. I'm always amazed at how many patients I see who don't know the side effects of the medicines they're taking. They are willing to put something into their bodies without being very clear about what it can do. I think most of them spend more time deciding about the clothes they wear than the medicines they take. I believe this happens because people do not listen to their doctors very well, and because sometimes doctors do not tell their patients very clearly what the side effects are of the medicines they prescribe. I have a simple approach. I do not give a patient a medicine until they understand just about as much about that medicine as I do.

A good example is amitriptyline. This is a very old antidepressant that was found to also act like an analgesic (pain killer). It is used all the time. It has a bunch of relatively minor side effects like dry eyes and mouth and constipation. It has some more concerning side effects like weight gain and sexual dysfunction. Finally, it has some deadly side effects. At high dose it can affect your heart rhythm and kill you. Make sure you understand what you are taking.

How Good Is the Research?

This is a complicated question and can be answered by people with a background in research. In order to understand how good research is you have to understand the research design and how to analyze research. However, it is not unreasonable to ask your doctor this question. They should be able to answer these questions. If your doctor cannot answer the questions, they should find the answers. If not, they shouldn't be prescribing the medicine and you shouldn't be taking it.

One more important point to make about medications. There are only three types of medicine:

1. Those that keep you alive. Insulin in diabetes is a perfect example of this. You can stop it if you like but you will suffer dire consequences.

2. Those that alter disease. Azathioprine (Imuran) is an immunosuppressant. I know because I take it. It keeps my disease under control. It does not cure it, but without it I am in big trouble. I stopped it once and three months later my entire right leg was paralyzed. I had horrific pain in my leg and I was being measured up for a wheelchair. Now, I never forget to take it even though it puts me at risk for certain cancers and problems with my liver.

3. The last type of medication is "everything else." Medications such as pain killers do not save lives or cure disease. They might make a person more comfortable. Nothing terrible will happen if you stop taking them. Whether you take them or not is a personal decision.

It's important to keep these ideas in mind because it will help you make intelligent decisions about whether to take a medicine for chronic pain. If you are diabetic, you have to take insulin or you could die. In the case of a drug like azathioprine, I learned the hard way that I had to take that drug or I'd be in deep trouble. In the case of pain meds, you won't die if you don't take them. Your pain might get worse, but your body does not need them to live. You therefore are in a position to make a clear decision about whether the supposed benefits of these medications outweigh the downside. You don't have to take them if you don't want to.

Now let's take a look at specific medicines used for the treatment of pain. There are a lot of medicines used to treat pain, too many to cover in a single chapter, so I will focus on those medicines that I think are important and that can teach us something of value. For over 20 years I have done a lecture in every pain group I have run about medication. I always start by simply asking people to tell me the names of medicines that they know about and I write down what they say on a blackboard. Usually the list contains more than 20 medicines. I try to group the medicines into specific families. The list has changed over time; two things seem to change it. First, new discoveries mean there are new medicines. Relatively recently a pain medicine called tramadol was introduced. Twenty years ago I would not have seen it on the list of medicines produced by patients, but I see it now. The other thing that affects the list is what's in and what's out. For example, 20 years ago I would never have seen opioids because physicians who used them for chronic pain were frowned upon. Now it is very common to see opioids on the list.

Let's take a look at a specific list of medicines used in pain management. Each of these medicines has a lesson to teach.

Opioids

Opioids are our most potent painkillers or analgesics. Opium is the basic medicine from which most narcotics or opioids spring. It is the dried latex of the opium poppy. There is evidence that its use dates back to Neolithic people. The Neolithic period starts at about 10,200 BCE. It was used by Sumerian, Assyrian, Egyptian, Indian, Minoan, Greek, Roman, Persian, and Arab empires for treating pain. By at least the 14th century opium was being used for recreational purposes in the Arab empire, and by the 15th century it was being used for the same purposes in China. Eventually it was mixed with tobacco and became more commonly abused, and by the 17th century the issue of addiction was recognized. What makes opium an interesting medicine is that it is the only medicine that is responsible for two wars. As you may remember, Great Britain went to war twice in the 19th century to make sure China kept buying the opium that the British were sending in from India so they could buy tea.

In 1804 Friedrich Sertürner isolated morphine from opium, allowing doctors to dose the medicine more specifically than they could with opium. From that point on, other opioids were synthesized. In 1874 heroin was synthesized by Bayer. Bayer sold it as an answer to morphine addiction. This is a very good example of what happens when you have poor research designs. As everyone knows, heroin is more addictive than morphine. Oxycodone was synthesized by Bayer in 1916. Methadone was synthesized in 1937 and fentanyl in the 1950s. We now have a host of options to choose from.

However, the next important question to ask, now that you understand the basis of pharmacology, is whether opioids actually work in treating chronic pain. Let's begin by asking a simple question: Do opioids reduce chronic pain?

In its recent guidelines, the Centers for Disease Control put it this way: "Evidence on long-term opioid therapy for chronic pain outside of end-of-life care remains limited, with insufficient evidence to determine long-term benefits versus no opioid therapy, though evidence suggests risk for serious harms that appears to be dose-dependent."

I went through some of the medical evidence about this question. There is some evidence that short-term use of opioids can help with pain. However, as we've already seen, they don't help everyone, and they don't erase the pain; they only make some people feel better. Here's the important thing for you to remember, though: *Long-term use does not seem very effective, and opioids seem to lose their efficacy with time.*

In my day-to-day practice, I am rarely impressed by how well these medications work. If you pick your patients carefully, choosing people who have no addiction problems and are very motivated to get moving, they can help. Unfortunately, more often than not I see people taking these medicines because they were told to, and all they are getting are side effects. The problem is, they are frightened about stopping them. They usually say, "If I stop them, what else will I take?" My response is "I have no idea but why would you take something that isn't working and that's causing you harm?"

Now let's ask the question in a different way: Do opioids reduce pain *and* improve function? In other words, do they help you get back to doing at least some of the things you like to do? As an expert on this issue, I've reviewed all the literature I can find on the performance of opioids, and I have yet to find any research evidence that tells me opioids alone significantly improve function in the majority of patients treated.

A very large epidemiological study was undertaken in Denmark. The group, led by Jorgen Erickson, a Danish anaesthetist, discovered that patients who were on long-term opioid therapy had higher levels of pain, had poorer quality of life, and were less functional than those patients who had chronic pain but were not being treated with long-term opioid therapy. This is very powerful research, but you need to remember that it does not show that the opioids actually caused these negative results. The negative side effects were associated with people who took opioids, but this does not mean that the opioids caused the negative side effects. Still, the results are worrisome, so as a doctor, I do everything possible not to use opioids. In fact, I spend more time taking people off them than putting them on opioids. Opioids are my last option and even then, not all the time.

So what are the risks of taking opioids?

Constipation

This side effect is extremely common. It's possible that up to 40 percent of patients will present with this problem. If left untreated, it can lead to bowel obstruction, which can become a surgical emergency. I know because it happened to my mother-in-law. Your doctor, then, should be asking you whether you have constipation. It's easy to handle, but dangerous if it's ignored.

Nausea, vomiting, and sweating

About 50 percent of people taking opioids feel nausea. Four percent vomit. Between 6 and 16 percent feel itchy and 34 percent have problems with sweating. We can stop the vomiting. In cancer treatment we use special medicines like Gravol and Stemetil to stop it, but using them for people with chronic pain makes little sense because those medicines will make you very tired and sleepy. The result is impaired function, not because of pain but because of the medicines you're taking. Whenever I see a patient on an antinausea drug, I review with them whether they are getting enough benefit from the opioid to make it all worthwhile. Some clinicians might use other medicines for the itching and sweating but these medicines cause their own problems. The itching and sweating come with the medicine and there is not a lot we can do about it.

Cognitive problems

Pain in and of itself affects people's cognitive ability but opioids make it worse.

An increase of pain

It's called opioid-induced hyperalgesia. Get ready for this. Taking opioids over a long period of time can actually lead to an increase in pain. It tends to be associated with some opioids more than others.

Low testosterone

A disorder called opioid-induced hypogonadism occurs more often in males. Put simply, being on long-term opioids can lead to the suppression of testosterone production. A man without testosterone is an ugly sight. No, you don't become more female. You become fat, lethargic, and asexual. I check the testosterone levels of every male in my clinic, and I find 6 out of 10 male patients who are taking opioids have low testosterone.

Addiction

This is what scares patients and physicians. Doctors regularly tell me that they refuse to prescribe opioids because of the risk of addiction and their fear that their college (the body that governs the behaviour of physicians) will take away their licence to practise if they do something wrong. My usual response is "Then go sell shoes" because these sorts of physicians should not be treating patients with chronic pain. To doctors I say: Learn how to do it and you have nothing to fear. It's that simple. At the very least, find someone who will handle prescribing this medicine responsibly if you cannot. Otherwise, the decision not to prescribe it is not about the patient's best interest, it's about your best interest.

One of the biggest problems is with the terms we use. People are fearful about addiction but it's not as common as you might think, in spite of the publicity about opioids. Anyone taking opioids for any length of time will be physically dependent on them and go into withdrawal if they stop taking the medicine. But they can be weaned off the medication, slowly, without terrible consequences. They are not psychologically dependent on it. They are not addicted to it.

Addiction occurs when a person is not only physically dependent on a substance but will do almost anything to get it, including lying and stealing. They are thinking about the drug all the time. This behaviour starts to affect their day-to-day lives. Such people often lose their jobs. They might take too much of the opioid—potentially lethal amounts—and they can't stop. They might engage in criminal activity to get the money to get the drug. These patients have a very high relapse rate with treatment. The draw of opioids is that it makes some people feel euphoric. I don't know what that feels like, but it must be great because people go through hell to feel it.

Another condition, pseudoaddiction, can look a lot like addiction. It occurs when a person takes more of an opioid than they were prescribed. They run out of the medicine early and try to get their doctor to prescribe more. This typically happens when a person's pain isn't controlled very well and they try to do something about it on their own. The patient starts using more medication than prescribed and might even borrow some from family or friends. They are trying to control their pain better. They also know their doctor will be upset if they admit that they used more than they should have, so they lie to try to get a prescription filled earlier than it should be. After all, because of their increased use of the opioid they ran out early. What is the treatment for this problem? The prescribing doctor needs to do a reassessment of the patient to determine if it is reasonable to increase their dose of opioids. Is there clear evidence that the medication, when used at higher doses than prescribed, improves function. If so, the dose should be increased. If not, help the patient withdraw from the opioid and think of an alternative treatment.

Physicians are understandably nervous about this medication. Most clinicians use a contract between the patient and doctor when using opioids. The contract outlines expectations and consequences for behaviour that could mean addiction. These behaviours include running out of medicine too soon or telling the doctor you lost your prescription so you need another one. Doctors want you to tell them the truth. Contracts spell out what will happen if these kinds of things happen. Usually a contract will state that no prescriptions will be given early . In this way if someone's pain is not well controlled on the dose they were given, they will talk with the doctor about it rather than self-medicating.

Another approach to deter overuse is urine testing. It can tell you whether certain medications like opioids and certain drugs like cocaine are present. This might help to identify someone who is abusing multiple substances or detect if a patient is not taking the opioid you prescribed but is diverting it because it is absent in the test. It does not, however, identify or diagnose opioid addiction or establish the presence of impairment or physical dependence.

The use of urine testing is controversial because of its limitations and what it means to many patients who feel they have done nothing wrong. In day-to-day pain management, I think urine testing provides very little in the way of helpful data. This testing does not tell me about addiction. I have yet to see research data demonstrating that urine testing reduces the risk of addiction or even opioid-related deaths, the worst outcome of opioid use. This test does tell the doctor about unsafe or bad behaviour. I do my best not to give these medications to any patient who makes me lose any sleep at all. I do not give them to patients using other substances. I work very hard at finding alternatives to opioids and, if I am going to prescribe them, screening my patients very carefully and monitoring them carefully. However, it is difficult to tell who is going to run into trouble with opioid therapy.

For some physicians, urine testing is perceived as helpful. Perhaps it is the nature of their patient population. However, what is important to note is that it is not a College requirement. In my role as an assessor for the College of Physicians and Surgeons of Ontario, I am told by countless physicians that they do urine testing because the College requires it. Not true. Know the facts about this test and then decide if it is helpful in your practice.

Look at me: I use these medicines. Over the years I have cut my dose in half. Why? In part because I hate the side effects. These medicines make me feel stupid. I can't remember things I did yesterday. The other reason is that the surgeon who fixed my back said to me, "No one ever gets off of narcotics and no one ever lowers their dose." He's wrong. I did. But these medicines make me constipated, nauseous, sweaty, and a bit stupid. I can assure you, I will never get addicted to them. As I said earlier, I don't even know what euphoria is. On the other hand, early in my career I treated a very pleasant man who was a bricklayer. He had a terrible fracture of his leg that ended his capacity to work. The only thing that gave him relief was opioids and he was one of the first patients I prescribed this medicine to. He was such a nice guy. As the years went by, he lost his prescriptions a couple of times and I refilled them. After all, he was a nice man. Once in a while he also ran out early and I helped him out there too. It was when he told me that a bird had flown into his car and taken his prescription that I knew something was very wrong. He confessed. He was addicted. The lesson for me was that addicts don't look all messed up, they look like you and me and it can happen to anyone.

How should doctors handle the danger of addiction? When I prescribe opioids, at my first follow-up I ask the patient an open-ended question: "How do you feel?" When someone responds, "It made me feel good (or great)," I ask a follow-up question: "How does it make you feel good?" If the patient says he feels good because his pain is settled, that's perfect. If he says he feels more relaxed, happier, and less upset, I start to wonder whether the patient has the brain for addiction. If he starts reporting that he has lost a prescription, or a friend stole some of his pills, it's a problem: there's a good chance that addiction has reared its head. That's when I start thinking about stopping the opioid.

The other thing I do is I give every patient a type of opioid addiction scale. These scales help to identify patients who are at high risk of addiction. Every new patient fills one of these scales out for me. If the result is high and there is a family or personal history of abuse, I try to steer far away from prescribing opioids. Sometimes a patient scores high but they have never abused a substance in their life. With these patients I think it is reasonable to begin a trial of opioids if required and monitor very carefully. You should be looking for reduced pain, improved function, and no evidence of euphoria or abuse. So the next time you think about using opioids to control your pain, remember a few interesting points:

- The evidence indicates that they do not help reduce pain very well and if they work, it is for a relative handful of people and for a short period of time.
- There are some serious side effects, including increased pain, and for men, low or no testosterone.
- Finally, there is a risk of abuse with opioids. I have a simple rule about this. I do not refill any prescription before it's time to do so, and if you start abusing the medication, I stop it.

One more point on the side effects: if opioids are used for a short term, less than three or four months, they cause no huge harm. That short-term use is quite uncommon to see in the chronic pain world, though, because most patients use these drugs for a long time and expect to be on them forever. Once a person is on them for a long period of time, they are at risk for harm. Look for other alternatives for pain control—like the self-hypnosis I will describe later in this book.

Gabapentinoids

Gabapentin was first approved for use in the United States in 1993. It was introduced as an antiseizure medicine. It is still used for mixed seizure disorders and refractory partial seizures in children and is a first-line treatment in the elderly who have seizures. It is used in focal lobe seizures not responsive to more typical first treatments.

Over time clinicians started to notice that gabapentin was very helpful for a certain type of pain called neuropathic pain, which comes from diseased or injured nerves and is one of the most difficult pains to have and to treat. At the time everyone thought it was a small miracle. Remember my "home run" burning mouth syndrome and how successful gabapentin was in that case. Clinicians in pain management started to use gabapentin for what is referred to as "off-label" use. This means we use the medicine for an indication not included in its licensing and has become a common practice in medicine. We started to use gabapentin for diseases of the nerves like diabetic neuropathy and post-herpetic neuralgia. It was very exciting—until recently. Now it appears that the NNT is about 4, which means 40 people have to take it so that 10 get 50 percent better. And here's the bad news: 6 out of 10 people have some kind of side effect, such as dizziness, weight gain, cognitive impairment, or swelling of the hands and feet. In other words, the cost benefit of this medication is not as good as we used to think. But that is not the main point here.

The next gabapentinoid was approved in 2004. It is called pregabalin—a chemical created by the liver when it tries to make gabapentin more water soluble so it can be eliminated from the body. Aren't you glad you know about pharmacokinetics? In other words, pregabalin is a metabolite of gabapentin, and for the most part works in exactly the same way.

But pregabalin, as the child of gabapentin, does one thing supremely well: because it's "new," it can be patented and the company can make profits from it. What's wrong with that? Just as gabapentin's patent comes to an end and the medication becomes generic, out comes pregabalin or Lyrica, its trade name. The company effectively is still making money from the original compound by using one of its metabolites that does not bring a lot of new things to the table.

This kind of behaviour is called "evergreening," and it's common in the pharmaceutical business these days. There are a lot of other medicines that are simple metabolites whose efficacy is typically not much better than the parent compound. They are usually not worth the cost to the patient but they make a lot of money for the pharmaceutical company.

NSAIDs

Nonsteroidal anti-inflammatory drugs (NSAIDs) have been around for a very long time and were partly responsible for the white man successfully landing in North America. We all remember Jacques Cartier, the French explorer who arrived on the Atlantic side of Canada in 1534. What some of us forget is that by the time he got to

North America, he and his entire crew were dying from scurvy, a lack of vitamin C. The natives of Canada knew what to do. They made a tea for Cartier and his crew from willow bark, a cure for scurvy and a source of salicylate, or what we now call aspirin. It was an early anti-inflammatory. The aboriginals did not know the pharmacology of willow bark, but they knew it cured certain illnesses.

How does any NSAID work? NSAIDs interrupt the inflammatory process by inhibiting an enzyme that is critical to the inflammatory response in the body. They are used for simple problems like a headache and more serious diseases like rheumatoid arthritis and lupus. They can also be used after a trauma because of inflammation from the injury. They can lower temperature so they are useful during fever. These medicines have tons of uses and are widely used, but they have a downside. By interfering with the inflammatory response, the older NSAIDs interfere with the stomach's ability to create the coating that protects it from its own acids. The result is ulcers created by the acid burning a hole in the stomach lining. This happens in 14.7 percent of patients.

The most common cause of an elderly person presenting to the emergency room vomiting blood is that they have been using an NSAID without taking anything to protect their stomach. Not a good thing. They have a bleeding ulcer that can be life threatening. In fact, the vast majority of people who take these medicines without some kind of stomach protection will develop gastritis, which is an inflamed wall of the stomach that pre-dates the ulcer, which is surely on its way.

Enter the COX-2 inhibitors, a type of NSAID. Celecoxib entered the market in North America in 1999. Then came others like rofecoxib that do pretty much the same thing. The difference is that they inhibit the enzyme involved in inflammation much more specifically than the old-time NSAIDs. They do not interfere with it in the stomach. Because of this they were supposed to be safer than the old time anti-inflammatories; people no longer had to worry about getting an ulcer. That was exciting news. Back in the day, *TIME* magazine put them on the cover under the headline "Super Aspirins." But now, many years later, we know better. Yes, they do not cause ulcers, but they can do something else that no one seemed to be aware of at the beginning. COX-2 inhibitors don't upset your stomach, but they can upset your heart.

The new danger was revealed by a large study in 2000 on rofecoxib. The study was looking into promising evidence that rofecoxib can shrink potentially cancerous polyps. When the study was done, five people out of the 1,287 taking robecoxib died of heart attack or stroke. In the group of 12,999 people taking a placebo, five people died. The real issue was the number of cardiac events. Twenty-five patients in the placebo group had these events compared to 45 people in the treatment group, a significant difference. Given the litigious world we live in, rofecoxib was pulled from the market and the recommended dose of celecoxib, the first COX-2 inhibitor, was controlled. Unfortunately this had a negative impact on many patients. A number of my patients with serious rheumatoid arthritis had very good pain control with rofecoxib, and since it has been taken off the market, I have found nothing else that works as well.

The lesson here is that sometimes we just don't know everything about a medication until it hits the market and is used by millions of people, instead of a few thousand in a clinical trial.

Amitriptyline and Cyclobenzaprine (Flexeril)

Amitriptyline was first identified as an antidepressant in the late 1930s and falls into the class of antidepressant called a tricyclic. It was discovered to be very useful for treating pain. In fact, this is one of the most common medications prescribed for chronic pain. It is an off-label use and one of the oldest off-label medications to be used for this purpose. It has been used for migraine headache, neuropathic pain, generalized pain, and almost every other painful condition you might think of. However, it comes with side effects. The medicine blocks a neuromodulator called acetylcholine. Don't worry what it is. By blocking it, you get at least 40 side effects, such as dry eyes, dry mouth, constipation, and sexual dysfunction. Sounds like fun. Still, the medication has been helpful to many patients for many years.

Cyclobenzaprine (Flexeril) is a medication that has also been used for many years to treat spasm, usually back spasm.

The number of patients I see taking both amitryptyline and Flexeril is huge. So what is wrong with that? The problem is Flexeril is also a tricyclic and has similar side effects to amitryptyline. By taking them together, you amplify the side effects. What's more, there's no evidence that taking them together produces extra pain relief. As far as I'm concerned, if you give patients both these drugs, you're double-dosing them and exponentially increasing the side effects. Why does this happen so frequently? Doctors don't know that they are from the same family of medications. No one told them in medical school. Most physicians actually believe Flexeril is an anti-spasmodic. Not quite. It is an analgesic just like amitriptyline.

Marijuana

Marijuana has gone from being an illegal recreational drug when I was a teenager to being so important that leaders of countries are making it part of their election platforms. It did not start out as a medication that has recreational value, like opioids. It started out as a recreational drug that found treatment value. Strange. It has also become a very common reason why a person is referred to me. I have been approached by companies that grow marijurana in the hopes that I will become, in effect, a "head" who directs people to buy the substance. That is why I won't do it, even though they do offer me an awful lot of money. I guess they make a lot and, therefore, so would I. Some patients bring me foods cooked with marijuana and even tincture of marijuana in order to help me feel better. I have never had any patient bring me morphine, but they will bring me marijuana. I don't use it, but it doesn't mean that a patient shouldn't. They need to treat it like any other medication.

Let's apply the same questions we've applied to other medications. Does it reduce pain? The answer is "Sort of." A series of studies by a scientist in Canada, Dr. M.A. Ware, has demonstrated that marijuana is better than placebo. That is certainly impressive.

However, it is not as simple as it looks. First, there is some criticism of Ware's research design. In a recent meta-analysis, it looked like marijuana appears to be helpful in the short term for neuropathic pain. Yet the volume of research and the study design were insufficient to draw a clear and absolute conclusion.

From where I sit, the research is insufficient to persuade me as a clinician and an expert on pain control in chronic pain patients that marijuana is very effective for the relief of chronic pain. The research focuses on pain reduction, not function. Here's another question: Is marijuana better than an opioid, an NSAID, or even acetaminophen? The truth is no one knows right now. I looked through the research data base used by medical researchers and found no evidence that marijuana for pain control has been tested against anything other than an inactive control, a placebo.

To date, no data compare the efficacy of marijuana to something as simple as an aspirin or Tylenol, let alone morphine. All the data say is that it appears to be better than taking absolutely nothing to reduce pain. Regarding the lack of data on function, I cannot tell a patient if they are better off taking an aspirin rather than using marijuana. So if you're going to use marijuana, you'd best be aware of its risks.

What about marijuana's side effects? Is smoking marijuana safe? Again the answer is yes and no. I see patients on a regular basis who have smoked marijuana most of their adult lives. They are now older and have a pain problem. It's not surprising that they would like to have their smoking of marijuana legitimized. They go on at great length about how incredibly safe marijuana is. There is only one problem. They have absolutely no background in science and so they don't know any of the facts, and they have a direct conflict of interest. They need it to be safe.

Make no mistake: marijuana smoke contains toxins. According to the American Lung Association (ALA), "Whether from burning wood, tobacco or marijuana, toxins and carcinogens are released from the combustion of materials. Smoke from marijuana combustion has been shown to contain many of the same toxins, irritants and carcinogens as tobacco smoke."

Marijuana smokers differ from tobacco smokers in two significant ways. They inhale more deeply and hold the smoke in longer, exposing the lung to tar longer. The ALA conclude that "clearly marijuana damages lung tissue." They note that smoking marijuana puts people who are HIV positive at increased risk of infection and there is a concern about infection with Aspergillus, a mould that grows on marijuana. This group cautions against the use of marijuana and is very concerned about second-hand inhalation.

There is good news, however. A very large international study was conducted looking at the risk of lung cancer in marijuana smokers. Guess what? There does not appear to be an increased risk in spite of the tar content.

The group concludes: "Results from our pooled analyses provide little evidence for an increased risk of lung cancer among habitual or long-term cannabis smokers, although the possibility of potential adverse effect for heavy consumption cannot be excluded." The reason for this is marijuana users tend to smoke a lot fewer joints compared to the number of cigarettes smoked by a cigarette smoker.

What about other side effects like fatigue, dizziness, and dry eyes? Lucky for us there is always a researcher around to answer an important question. The result is a large study called the COMPASS study. It looked at this very question in 215 people, current users and ex-users. They found that although people who used marijuana had more side effects than people not using marijuana, they were not serious side effects. They conclude, "Quality-controlled herbal cannabis, when used by patients with experience of cannabis use as part of a monitored treatment program over 1 year, appears to have a reasonable safety profile. Longer-term monitoring for functional outcomes is needed."

These researchers tell us that marijuana use is benign for the most part. But the story is not that simple. Another set of researchers tells us that there is risk attached to its use. A Canadian epidemiological study of thousands of people taking marijuana in 2012 showed that 55,813 years of life were lost due to disability caused by the use of marijuana. The typical disability identified was death, cannabis use disorders (psychiatric illness), schizophrenia, lung cancer, and road traffic injuries. The authors also note that the number of years lost in this group of marijuana smokers is less than that typically seen in other commonly used legal and illegal substances. So, if you are going to use marijuana, contrary to my patient who would like to believe otherwise, there is some risk attached.

In my experience, it's the old-time marijuana smoker who reaches for marijuana to control chronic pain—not people who have not used the substance ever or for many years. The research suggests that it's safer for experienced users to smoke dope to kill pain than it is for inexperienced ones.

There is one serious side effect that is worth mentioning: psychosis in younger people. Psychosis can lead to serious perceptual disturbances like hearing voices saying very negative things to a patient. Imagine that going on all day long. This is a very serious illness. The vast majority of patients and physicians do not seem to be aware of this side effect of marijuana. Psychosis can be precipitated by marijuana in a vulnerable person. The real problem is we have no way of knowing who is vulnerable until this terrible side effect occurs. It was found that the more a person uses marijuana, the higher the risk. However, the association is not an absolute and the side effect is not common. We always need more research to firm up our findings, but the phenomenon exists and it destroys lives.

Conclusion

Using medicines is a serious business. The vast majority of medicines used in pain management have serious side effects, so you have to ask yourself whether it's worth taking them. These are not medicines that keep you alive or alter the course of your disease. They are medicines that help to manage a problem, and if you stop them, nothing bad will happen, other than the potential for more pain. If you use medicines, make sure you know their negative side effects, and make a clear decision whether they are working for you, and whether the negative side effects are worth it.

5

Discovering
Hypnosis

At 29, I was working as a social worker at a large hospital for very troubled children. By this point my back and right leg were killing me, every day. I had not had any surgery as yet. I had seen physicians all over Ontario and got a wide variety of recommendations. Some told me to do exercise. Unfortunately some of the exercises that they recommended, I could not do. They made my pain much worse. One surgeon tried to give me morphine. Thirty years ago that was uncommon and I said no thank you. Others suggested surgery but none of them agreed on the type of surgery. The whole process did not inspire confidence. Besides, I could still walk and stand independently. I was not ready for surgery. The only problem I had was that I had pain all day long. By the end of the day my pain was worse. It was unrelenting. It would not let up. It just ground away at me and was slowly eroding my life.

Even after my back and leg pain got bad, I still played tennis. I swam 40 lengths three times a week and I weight-lifted. I was 140 pounds and bench-pressed 225 pounds. Fat lot of good it did me. As the pain got worse, I started doing less and less. The tennis stopped. The swimming reduced, and the weightlifting disappeared. My six pack became a four pack and slowly eroded to a single pack. I was becoming less energetic and, frankly, boring to be around.

I was taking no medicine. I had nothing to control my pain. Then a friend of mine, another social worker where I worked, invited me to a group he was part of. It was a hypnotherapy group. At that time social workers were not allowed to do hypnosis so I felt like I was part of an underground group. It seemed so cool at the time. I remember my first meeting like it was yesterday.

The meeting took place at the facility where we worked. We were in an interview room so there was a one-way mirror, although no one was watching us from behind it. Everyone looked pretty odd. They were all doing various incantations and mumbling at each other. It took me a while to understand what was going on. It was simply a disorganized group of health care providers who had an interest in hypnosis. To the uninformed like me, it simply looked silly. People were trying various hypnotic inductions on each other, but it was done in a disorganized manner. (We call it induction because it is a word everyone is familiar with—it simply means someone is going into a trance.)

I kept going to these meetings in spite of the fact that I had no idea what was really going on because I had no other choice and this was not going to do me any harm. I could leave any time I wanted to. Eventually someone suggested a more organized approach, and the group started doing one induction at a time. They understood there were some people like me who knew nothing about hypnosis, so they started to teach me how to do it. Eventually I got a reasonable understanding of what a hypnotic induction was. The only problem was, it seemed that I could not be hypnotized.

Each time the group met, someone would do a new induction and someone would volunteer to be the subject. Afterward we would all go home and practise what we'd seen. The intent was we would learn how to hypnotize ourselves. For me, it never happened. I never went into a trance even though I really wanted to. I was never able to hypnotize myself and I really did practise almost every day.

I avoided volunteering in the group like poison. Not because I was fearful but because I did not want the would-be hypnotist to feel bad. However, eventually my number was up. There were about 15 of us and everyone had already volunteered. I had even done an induction in front of this group, and my subject had gone into a very profound trance. It was now my turn to be that subject. The hypnotist did his thing. I thought he was quite good at it. I even closed my eyes for him. At the end of his incantation, he tested me for hypnotic phenomena—dissociation, time distortion, or even just feeling very relaxed. There was nothing there. I was not hypnotized. I felt very bad about it. Like I said, I am not a very good hypnotic subject.

The group piqued my interest but I knew there was a lot more to learn. I travelled around North America working with some of the top hypnotists of the 1980s. Unfortunately, I would not go into a trance for these hypnotherapists either even though they were the best of the best. I learned their methods but I would not go into a trance. I never got any pain control out of the deal. It was not because I didn't want to—I desperately wanted to be hypnotized or to hypnotize myself. Unfortunately I am just one of those people who are poor subjects.

In spite of this liability, I did not give up. I still had no other reasonable option and my pain was terrible. I had learned about as much as I was going to about hypnosis. I knew how to do clinical hypnosis. I even knew how to do stage hypnosis. I could hypnotize someone else but I just couldn't hypnotize myself. I decided to dedicate myself to the process of putting myself into a trance.

I practised diligently. I did it almost every day for about half an hour. I just kept at it for almost a year. Then one day, out of the blue, I did it. I put myself into a trance. How did I know I'd been successful? I'd gone through my usual induction process. Suddenly, I felt like I was floating well above where I was sitting. Then everything turned black even though I thought my eyes were open and the room was well lit. I saw multiple sets of eyes looking at me. Honest. I didn't feel frightened because I knew I had done this on my own. Nor did I think some bizarre metaphysical event was occurring. I thought that the whole thing was weird but I was determined to hang in there with it for as long as I could. It felt like hours before the eyes disappeared and the lights in the room returned. In fact it was only 15 minutes. This was my first trance, and I proved I was in a trance because I was experiencing a hypnotic phenomenon. That sense of time being longer than it really is is called time dilation. This was proof of trance.

So now what? I now knew I could put myself into a trance. That seemed pretty important. Maybe I could put myself into a trance and control my pain also. Isn't that why I was doing this in the first place? So I started practising my trance and now I included one of the pain control methods I'd learned. The first time I did this I got a 10 percent reduction in my pain. For me it was a miracle. To that point, nothing had improved my pain, absolutely nothing. I now did the process every day. As the months went by, my skills improved and my pain reduction increased. At times I got 30 percent reduction. At the very least I got 10 percent improvement. To this day I have not found a medicine that works better. I went on to study with a number of recognized experts in hypnosis. Each had their own style. I learned from more authoritarian style hypnotherapists and from Ericksonian hypnotherapists (more about Erickson and his methods in the next chapter). Each brought something unique to the table. I learned a great deal from these people. I learned that hypnosis is not induced even though we call putting someone into a trance an induction, as mentioned earlier. In fact, we elicit the trance phenomena. We set a stage so people go into a trance rather than forcing or inducing them to do it. I also learned to respect the various styles of hypnosis. What is important to remember is that to date there is no scientific evidence that makes one method of hypnosis better than another.

As the years have gone by, my professional career has expanded. I went on to be trained as a physician, psychiatrist, and finally a pain specialist. As a pain specialist, I was now in a perfect position to pass on to patients what I had taught myself. I put together a hypnotherapy group and began teaching patients how to do self-hypnosis for pain control. This group has been very successful over the years. The vast majority of patients reduce their pain and some reduce their reliance on opioid medications. That is amazing.

For me, I still use self-hypnosis for pain control every day. I have gotten much faster at it and I need less formal induction to get to a point where I can control my pain. However, I have never been able to get more than 30 percent reduction in pain. I have patients who get close to 100 percent reduction in pain although they tend to be much better subjects than me.

In spite of these impressive results, most of my colleagues in the medical community haven't picked up on the news. In fact, last year I was scheduled to present a seminar series for doctors on this subject. Only one person signed up. Doctors, especially family physicians, treat plenty of patients for chronic pain, and as we've seen, they're grappling with the serious problems that accompany opioid use. So why don't they want to learn how to do hypnosis or, at the very least, recommend it? It has no side effects, and as we'll see, there's growing proof that it works. Yet, as far as I know, I am the only physician in my entire community who teaches these skills to patients. I am also the only person I know, other than the patients I have taught, who uses this skill to manage pain.

So where does the resistance come from? I think the answer may lie in the curious history of hypnosis and the beliefs my colleagues have about what hypnosis is all about. Let's look at the history of hypnosis in the next chapter.

6

History of
Hypnosis

Hypnosis has a long, and fascinating history—both as a medical tool and as a source of public entertainment. When you hear the story, you'll understand why clinicians and patients with pain might be reluctant to take advantage of this clinical tool, in spite of scientific evidence that it can help reduce chronic pain.

The use of trance dates back to about 3000 BCE in ancient Persia and India, where it was used in a religious context to treat the sick. It's been used all over the world by religious sects, like the Cabalists of Judaism, the Christian Firewalkers of Greece, the Taoists of East Asia, the Yogis of Sufi Hinduism, and the Whirling Dervishes of Sunni Islam. They used it to heal and whip up a religious fervour in their devotees. In 1000 AD, the Persian physician

Avicenna, or IbnSīnā, used trance to heal the sick during the golden age of Islam.

With time, however, the practice of trance induction acquired props. In the 1600s, Valentine Greatrakes induced trance while passing magnets over the sick. He was a religious man who truly believed he had a God-given gift to cure by driving evil out of people. A century later, magnets became associated with trance induction. In the mid-1700s, a Viennese Jesuit, Father Maximilian Hell, applied magnets attached to steel plates to the naked bodies of his subjects.

Hell's protégé, Franz Anton Mesmer, was one of the most important names in the history of hypnosis. Mesmer's name lives on in the word "mesmerize," which means to hold someone as if they were in a spell. Mesmer, working in the mid- to late 18th century, disposed of the magnets and relied instead on his own innate "animal magnetism," a term he coined. He also created the Mesmeric Pass, the passage of his hands over the affected person. Mesmer believed that there was some kind of an invisible force, "magnetic fluids," in animals of all kinds that could exert physical effects on other animals, including the power to heal. He would use his own "animal magnetism" to "cure" the ill. His work gained popularity throughout Europe. He performed his cures one on one or in front of groups. Sitting across from his subjects with his knees touching theirs, he would press their thumbs into his hands. He would pass his hands over the person and then press his fingers into an area of the body referred to as the hypochondrium, an area just under the rib cage. Sometimes he would hold his hands in this area for hours at a time. Once he finished his treatment, he would then play an unusual instrument called a glass armonium. The whole procedure was a mix of healing and entertainment.

Mesmer eventually moved from Vienna to Paris, the intellectual capital of its time. He gathered a large group of followers around him, made up of the upper class and court nobility. The group included Wolfgang Amadeus Mozart and the Queen of France, Marie Antoinette. He held large group sessions, moving around a darkly lit room, passing his hands over his followers in order to channel his magnetic fluids to them. He became quite a celebrity in Paris although the Queen's husband, Louis XVI, was not one of his fans. Because Louis thought Mesmer was a quack, he gathered together a group of intellectuals from France's Royal Academy of Science to investigate Mesmer's claims. This group included such famous personalities as the mayor of Paris, Jean Bailly; Dr. Joseph-Ignatius Guillotin, the inventor of the instrument that would eventually end the lives of Louis XVI and the Queen; the astronomer, mathematician, and later French Revolutionary, Jean Sylvain Bailly; and Benjamin Franklin, the great American statesman. The tests were conducted at Franklin's home in Passy. Rather than appearing before the committee, Mesmer sent a representative, Dr. Charles Deslon. If everything went well, Mesmer would take the credit. If things went badly, Mesmer could blame Deslon.

Franklin and his colleagues devised what is now considered the first control trial ever documented. The experiment was relatively simple by today's standards. Blindfolded patients were shown to respond to a non-magnetized tree as if it had been imbued with Mesmer's animal magnetism, as well as to one that was magnetized by Mesmer's methods. The committee concluded that "the imagination without the magnetism produces convulsions, and the magnetism without the imagination produces nothing."

This was, amazingly, considered the first recorded control trial in the history of research.

Mesmer left Paris, a debunked charlatan. But the commission's work had the opposite effect than intended. It provided Mesmer with a great deal of free publicity and Mesmerism continued to be practised for another century with a brief revival in Victorian England, long after Mesmer died in Germany in 1815.

In spite of the negative press associated with Mesmerism, the belief in animal magnetism, along with the use of magnets and the Mesmeric Pass, persisted. A critical figure at this time was the Indo-Portuguese monk, Abbé Faria. He practised in the late 18th and early 19th centuries. He made a significant contribution to the development of clinical hypnosis by stripping animal magnetism, the use of magnets, and the Mesmeric Pass from hypnosis. He developed a form of hypnosis we would recognize in clinical settings today. He postulated that hypnosis worked purely by suggestion. An early client-centred therapist, he concluded that nothing came from the magnetizer and everything came from the imagination and mind of subject. He was the first to apply what would now be termed scientific methodology to the practice of hypnosis and had a significant influence on hypnosis in the late 19th century.

Hypnosis eventually found its way into the operating room. By the time Mesmer made hypnosis popular, surgery had come a long way from the feared barber-surgeons of the Middle Ages. Surgery was still frightening, though. Anaesthesia had not been discovered yet, and even minor procedures could be lethal because of rampant infection. The most common surgical procedure was amputation. Unlike today when the patient is anaesthetized throughout the procedure, the patient, screaming as their limb was sawed off, would be held down by medical assistants.

Then a 19th-century Scottish surgeon, James Braid, attended a session run by a mesmerist named Charles Lafontaine. Lafontaine was probably the first big stage hypnotist who toured Britain with his act. At first Braid was quite cynical about hypnosis. However, he returned a second time and was struck by a hypnotic phenomenon called eye cataplexy, in which the subject is unable to open their eyes under hypnotic trance. Braid, along with colleagues, including a prominent eye surgeon, mounted the stage during the act when a female subject was in trance and displaying eye cataplexy. When the physicians raised the girl's closed eyelids, the pupils were constricted, an involuntary act that they interpreted as meaning that the girl was in deep sleep. Braid then jammed a pin under the girl's fingernail. She was unresponsive, completely anaesthetized. Braid was impressed. He returned to Lafontaine's act three more times to observe his methods. He learned how to do hypnosis and started to practise it on his patients. He discovered that he could induce trance in patients without all the Mesmeric rigmarole and recognized the potential of hypnosis as a method for pain control during his surgeries. He saw that the results of the Mesmeric Pass really came from the subject paying very close attention to some brightly moving object or some object upon which they fixated, a method still used today. The classic pocket watch swinging back and forth in front of the hypnotic subject can be attributed to James Braid.

It was James Braid who first coined the term "hypnosis," which comes from the late Latin word *hypnoticus* meaning to "induce sleep." The word was first coined in 1841 and first used in an unpublished essay by Braid called "Practical Essay on the Curative Agency of Neurohypnotism (1842)". Eventually Braid concluded that hypnosis is not a state of sleep, which is true, and he tried to change the name to "monoideism," which means a "preoccupation with a single thing or idea," but it was already too late—the term hypnotism had caught on.

In 1846, ether was used for the first time to put surgical patients to sleep and thereby control pain. Surgery was changed forever, and surgeons moved away from hypnosis as a method of pain control during surgical treatments. Although hypnosis was still used for painful problems that could not be fixed by surgery, clinical hypnotherapists turned their primary attention from surgical pain control to the treatment of psychological problems. This shift led, through a number of pathways running through France, to the father of psychoanalysis, Sigmund Freud. Freud was deeply influenced by 19th-century French thinking on hypnosis and even translated a book by Hippolyte Bernheim, a French neurologist who investigated the power of suggestion, into German.

There were two important schools of hypnotic thought in France in the 19th century. One was the Salpêtrière School, or Paris school, under the revered physician Jean-Martin Charcot, the founder of modern-day neurology. One of Charcot's topics of research was hysteria, an anachronistic term, no longer in clinical use. It was used to describe patients who, as a result of overwhelming fear of some past traumatic event, focused that fear on a body part instead of facing the fear. This could result in paralysis without evidence of any neurologic disorder or people forgetting long periods of time only to find out that they behaved like a different person during these episodes. Although seen less frequently today than in the late 19th century, patients still present with "hysterical paralysis" or what is now called conversion disorder and unusual changes in personality or "dissociation." Up to this time, hysteria was thought to have physiologic causes. Charcot was the first physician of substance to postulate that it was a psychological illness. He believed hypnotizability represented an abnormality found in patients with this disorder. Hypnosis allowed patients with hysteria to uncover childhood fears and trauma. He then used this finding to postulate that trauma of the past led to the symptoms of hysteria in the present. Charcot presented his work to the medical community, where it was accepted as a legitimate theory.

Chacot's theories were soon challenged by a rival, the Nancy School, located in the French town of Nancy. Its leader, Ambroise-Auguste Liébeault saw hypnosis as "induced sleep," produced by the suggestion of sleep within an atmosphere of rapport with the hypnotherapist. He thought anyone could be hypnotized, that it was a normal attribute found in varying degrees in everyone. At the time of the Nancy School's initial publications, it was Charcot's work that still held sway, but a few years later, in the early 20th century, the Nancy School won the psychological war. Over time, Liébeault's views have had a lasting impact on the field of hypnotherapy. He influenced neurologist Hippolyte Bernheim, who introduced hypnotherapy to a wider medical audience, including Sigmund Freud.

Freud was a student of Charcot's and was greatly influenced by his work in hysteria. He was also aware of the theories of the Nancy School. However, it was Charcot's influence that gained the upper hand in Freud and can be seen in Freud's work with hysterical paralysis. Charcot's concepts helped Freud develop his concept of the unconscious mind, in which powerful mental processes were hidden from the conscious awareness of the individual.

Freud used hypnotism as a tool during his first years of practice, putting his patients into a trance in order to uncover past trauma. He would have his patients fix their eyes on two of his fingers while the patient paid attention to any bodily sensations that developed. At that time he believed that not only was hysteria accessible through hypnosis but so were the symptoms of other organic disorders. It was through his use of hypnotherapy that Freud came to appreciate that there are many painful memories repressed or forgotten in the unconscious mind, a psychological process designed to protect a person from psychological pain. This led to his concept of the unconscious mind. He came to believe that the behaviour of patients following post-hypnotic suggestion was proof of the unconscious mind. However, he became concerned that patients would become addicted to the hypnotic process like a narcotic and lose touch with the present situation. Also, Freud, who some scholars consider a beginner as a hypnotherapist, was unable to put all patients into a useful therapeutic trance.

After Freud abandoned hypnotherapy, hypnosis was still practised by some clinicians. Yale researcher Clark Hull even tried to give it a scientific basis in his 1933 book, *Hypnosis and Suggestibility*. Nonetheless, there were growing fears about hypnosis. Canadian-American psychologist George Estabrooks claimed to have been called in by the American military during World War II to use hypnosis for the benefit of the allies. He claimed that hypnosis could be used to completely control another person's behaviour. He painted the frightening picture of enemy agents being embedded in the United States, perhaps posing as physicians on military bases. Through their use of hypnosis, they could take over the entire base. A lowly lieutenant could be hypnotized by a saboteur to become the perfect weapon, taking over the military establishment. Estabrooks boasted that he could create an army of saboteurs to fight the enemy and bragged that he could hypnotize American citizens to commit treason against the U.S. government. He believed that hypnosis could be dangerous and that contrary to the attitude of the majority of hypnotherapists that a subject cannot be induced to do something they find morally wrong, this psychologist stated emphatically that it was not up to the subject of hypnosis, but the hypnotist. A hypnotist could make a person do anything he wanted.

This fear of the power of hypnosis did not end with Estabrooks. The flame was fanned by John G. Watkins, an American psychologist. He and his wife developed a form of treatment, still in use in some centres today, called "ego-state therapy." This treatment aimed to uncover underlying personalities to deal with psychological problems. Watkins said he even elicited a confession from a murderer this way. Watkins performed a series of experiments in 1947 during which he hypnotized normal young soldiers to believe that their officer was a Japanese soldier intent on killing them. In these experiments, the hypnotized soldier would leap up and try to strangle the officer, believing that it was a case of life or death. In one experiment, the subject had a hidden knife. Fortunately, he was disarmed.

The story of mind control and hypnosis does not end here. There is the famous case in Denmark of Palle Hardrup and Bjorn Nielsen that took place in the 1950s. Hardrup was a young man who made the mistake of joining the Nazi party four months before the Allies arrived. He was then sent to prison by the Allies, where he met Nielsen, a petty criminal and con artist. Eventually Nielsen induced Hardrup to commit robberies, supposedly under hypnotic influence. Hardrup claimed that while in trance he believed he was committing these crimes for nationalistic purposes. Unfortunately, one of the robberies went very wrong and he killed a teller and bank manager. Ultimately, Nielsen and Hardrup came to trial. People who had previously been in jail with Hardrup and Nielsen reported that Hardrup was completely under the control of Nielsen. It was later reported that the hypnotic signal was an X, and Nielsen would sit in front of Hardrup during the trial, with his legs or arms crossed, supposedly influencing the young man's statements. Eventually, both were found guilty. Hardrup was committed to an institution for the criminally insane. Nielsen spent some time in jail but eventually won his release through the appeals process.

Since these events there has always been an underlying fear by the general public that hypnotists can control the minds of people. They'd think of Bela Lugosi's version of Count Dracula in the 1931 horror classic when he induces a victim to come to him with the command "Come to me," repeated over and over.

Hypnotism was revived as a stage act in the 1940s, when Ormond McGill's book, *The Encyclopaedia of Genuine Stage Hypnotism*, became the bible of the trade. By then the image of the all-powerful hypnotist who could induce people to do just about anything was firmly entrenched in the minds of many Americans. An American stage hypnotist, Ralph Slater, was sued by a woman claiming that she had been damaged by his show. Although the case against Slater was not successful, it led to the 1952 Hypnotism Act in Britain, which was designed to regulate the behaviour of stage hypnotists. Given that most people think of stage hypnosis when they think of hypnosis, is it any wonder that people are somewhat reluctant to think of hypnosis for the clinical treatment of pain.

The father of modern-day clinical hypnosis, Milton Erickson, was one of the most gifted hypnotherapists in history. He was both dyslexic and profoundly colour blind. He had multiple "autohypnotic" experiences while recovering from severe polio. He would suddenly go into a trance-like state. For a time he was unable to speak because of his disease, leading him to acquire advanced skills in the ability to observe body language and paralanguage, the meaning of a person's tone of voice. It was from these experiences that Erickson developed his unique approach to hypnosis. His work came to the attention of the general public through Jay Haley's 1973 book, *Uncommon Therapy*. I was fortunate enough to be a student of Haley's.

Erickson believed that the unconscious mind is always present and that successful hypnotic suggestions can be made as long as they are acceptable to the unconscious mind. He also believed that trance was a common human phenomenon, such as daydreaming. The hypnotherapist is simply taking advantage of these common trance states. The patient might or might not be aware of what was happening. There were times when Erickson would go into trance along with his subjects, believing that this improved the therapist's ability to resonate with the patient.

Erickson developed a naturalistic method of hypnosis—this is different from the classic authoritarian style of hypnosis. The authoritarian hypnotherapist might say, "You will now go into a deep trance" while the naturalistic hypnotist would say, "If you allow yourself to notice the rhythmic nature of your breathing, you might also notice that with each breath in you become more relaxed." Erickson would take advantage of the natural physical rhythms of his patients. He believed that the unconscious mind could not be directed through conscious pathways, it had to be opened up through trance. He also believed that authoritarian styles of hypnosis led the unconscious mind to resist suggestion while naturalistic methods led the unconscious to be more open to suggestion. Erickson went on to develop a number of methods of trance induction. He would intentionally confuse a patient to put him into a trance, or he might shake a person's hand, but then suddenly grab their wrist, again inducing a trance. These techniques are still used by some clinicians today, although there's no evidence that they work any better than any other style of hypnosis.

At times hypnosis has been seen as a useful clinical tool, while at other times, it's been seen as a tool that can be used to manipulate the minds of others—sometimes for the amusement of hundreds of people in the audience. Unfortunately, the image of hypnosis as a tool to control minds for nefarious purposes is still a powerful one, even though there's no evidence that clinicians have used it this way. Current research, as we will soon see, has demonstrated a useful clinical effect of hypnosis in the management of chronic pain. Yet all too often, people are reluctant to try it because they fear they will do something they don't want to do. They think they'll be the unfortunate subject of some kind of stunt. They needn't worry in a health care setting. We have to remember that hypnotherapy, by definition, is used by trained professionals to help people in need of assistance. All physicians have taken the Hippocratic oath, which requires that physicians "do no harm" to their patients. If the patient trusts a surgeon who uses a scalpel, a tool that can cause untold harm in the wrong hands, they should trust trained hypnotherapists who have an ethical obligation to act in the best interest of their patient.

Now let us take a look at the research literature on hypnotherapy. Does it work? Is there evidence that it can help you and me control our pain? How does hypnosis work?

7

The Science Behind Hypnosis: Does It Work? How?

H ypnosis has a long and storied history in medicine and on the stage. But the question you might ask is this: How does it work? Is there research evidence that it works to control pain? I know it's worked for me, and I've seen it work for my patients. But that's not a sufficient proof. How can we prove it works? To explore the question, let's begin by asking what hypnosis is.

The best definition I've found comes from a textbook by David Spiegel and Jose Maldonado, professors at Stanford University: Hypnosis is a natural state of aroused, attentive focal concentration with relative suspension of peripheral awareness. It involves an intensity of focus that allows the hypnotized person to make maximal use of innate abilities to control perception, memory, and somatic function.

The way I think of it is a bit simpler. Hypnosis is a state of narrowed attention to one's internal state. In this state a person can gain better control over their own natural abilities to control pain.

When most people think of hypnosis, they're thinking of stage hypnosis—when a hypnotist finds a subject, does a very dramatic induction, and the person falls into a deep trance. They are then asked to do something unusual like think they are a chicken and the person starts clucking. Although entertaining this has nothing to do with clinical hypnosis.

One of the key features of stage hypnosis is *suggestibility*. Suggestibility means that a person accepts what is said without volition or choice. The normal emotional, social, and intellectual critical filters are shut off. It is like almost any other human characteristic. Some people have a lot, and some have a little, with most people being somewhere in the middle.

For the stage hypnotist, a critical part of the job is finding good subjects—people who are most likely to follow the hypnotist's suggestions with the understanding that these suggestions will not be harmful and the entire process is meant to be enjoyable. That's why the stage hypnotist typically comes out before the performance begins and goes through a series of exercises with the audience. He's looking for the candidates who are suggestible and can help him create an entertaining performance.

Scientific researchers have even devised a way to test how suggestible a person is. It's the Stanford Hypnotic

Susceptibility Scale, developed in 1959. The tester reads out some small hypnotic inductions and the subject measures how deeply they felt what was being suggested. If the tester asks the subject to imagine putting his hand in very cold water, the subject then measures on a 10-point scale how cold his hand actually felt. It's far from perfect, but it is the most commonly used test of suggestibility.[1]

Highly suggestible people are great subjects for stage hypnotism, and, based on my observations, they tend to learn how to do self-hypnosis more quickly and to get better results. I can see that in one of my patients, Peter, who is very suggestible. He learned how to do self-hypnosis very quickly and he gets very good pain control. I am not as suggestible, it took me a long time to learn how to do self-hypnosis, and my pain control is less than his. Suggestibility varies by sex and age. It appears to be higher in women. It also appears to decrease between the ages of 17 and 40 and then increase again.

However, in clinical hypnosis, suggestibility is not central. In my work I do not care how suggestible a person is. My focus is on teaching the person a method for controlling pain. The person is not there for my entertainment, and I do not ask them to do anything other than learn how to use hypnosis to reduce their pain. It is not nearly as much fun to watch as stage hypnosis, but it can play an important role in helping someone live a better life.

So how does hypnosis in clinical practice work? There are a number of theories about this. One is the state theory, which is based on the idea that hypnosis is a *physiologic* phenomenon.[2] Something changes in the person's physiology. For example, one theory suggests that the frontal lobe, which is responsible for our executive function and judgment, "gives up" and becomes functionally impaired in a hypnotic state. Some research evidence shows that hypnosis is associated with changes in the brain.

To back up the state theory, there's a significant amount of data involving imaging in the form of either positron emission tomography (PET) or functional magnetic resonance imaging (fMRI), and the measurement of brain activity using electroencephalograms (EEG). The findings have been varying and sometimes contradictory, but in the big picture, what we learn is that something seems to happen when a person goes into trance that can be demonstrated using these tools.[3]

One intriguing bit of evidence supporting the idea that hypnosis causes a physiologic change comes from a case study by Dr. Peter Halligan and colleagues at a university in Wales.[4] Although case studies are considered weak in the world of research, they tend to be easy to understand and often point the way to future research. These researchers were interested in the psychiatric illness called conversion. In conversion a person might have a paralyzed limb, although there are no physical reasons for this. However, they are not faking, so it is thought that psychological factors are at play. This illness was central to the work of Sigmund Freud. Halligan compared the PET scan results of a suggestible, physically well subject who was hypnotized. In that state he was given the suggestion that he had a paralyzed leg. The PET scan of this subject, while in trance and experiencing paralysis, was compared with a colleague's PET scan of a patient who had paralysis of a leg as a result of a conversion disorder. The scans were surprisingly similar. Although there can be other reasons for the similarity in scan results, the result is interesting.

The other group of theories are referred to as non-state theories. They focus more on how the person's psychological state of mind and their environment sets the stage for them to fall into a trance. According to this theory, hypnosis offers the person a chance for pain relief and because of this, they expect a positive result when they go into a trance. It's similar to responding to a placebo medication—when a person is given a placebo medication but is told that it is a powerful painkiller. If they use it for a headache, the likelihood that their headache reduces is increased.[5]

The most common question is this: "Isn't hypnosis just a placebo?" The answer is yes and no. Both hypnosis and placebo can result in analgesia in the right subject. They both have an impact on the somatosensory network of the brain. However, they are also different. There is evidence that placebo responses can be associated with physiologic changes in the limbic (emotional) structures of the brain. Hypnotic pain relief seems to have a higher association with changes in the occipital, or visual, areas of the brain.

The placebo response is mediated by opioids that are inside humans, the endogenous opioids. So to answer the question of whether hypnosis acts like a placebo, one group of researchers conducted a test. They induced hypnotic analgesia and then blocked opioid receptors in the body by using the medicine naloxone. Naloxone is the same medicine used when a patient has had an overdose of opioids. If hypnosis did act like a placebo, the effects of hypnosis would be reversed by the naloxone , which can block some placebo responses. When researchers conducted the experiment, they discovered that naloxone did not change the effects of hypnotic analgesia. This was a significant finding. It reinforces the point that hypnosis is not simply a placebo.

Researchers now suggest hypnosis has an impact. According to one European study, the analgesic effect of hypnosis on acute produced pain (typical experimental methods of inducing pain) is "probably more than just placebo effect in terms of brain functionality."

The real issue for me and my patients, though, is whether hypnosis is a proven pain reliever. Although by nature I am an academic thinker who is not easily sold on something because I am told it is good, in the case of hypnosis I know that it works for me. I can usually reduce my pain by about 20 to 30 percent. As I said earlier, I have never achieved better results. My patient Peter can achieve close to 100 percent relief and as a result he has reduced his use of opioid medications. So, between Peter and me there is case-based evidence that hypnotherapy can reduce chronic pain. Unfortunately, case-based data are just about the weakest form of research data there are. So what does the medical research say about the impact of hypnosis on pain?

When I started my search into the medical literature about hypnosis and chronic pain, I began by looking at the literature on acute pain first. After all, acute pain should be easier to manage. Acute pain is pain that more often than not arises out of some trauma and it is expected to go away once the trauma heals. A good example is a fractured bone. This is not pain that has been present for months and years. Significant research exists on this topic looking at a variety of areas of medical practice. Hypnosis has been shown to be helpful in reducing pain in such problems as burn care, post-operative pain, chemotherapy/radiation induced pain, bone marrow aspiration in adults and children, invasive medical procedures in adults and children, and even labour. Overall, hypnosis has a positive impact on acute pain. It might not be perfect, relieving all the problems associated with these medical issues, but it does help.

What evidence is there that hypnosis helps to manage chronic pain? Other than my say-so, and that of Peter's, is there any scientific evidence that hypnosis can help control chronic pain?

The results for acute pain mean very little for chronic pain, because, as we have seen, chronic pain lasts a lifetime and can have a profound effect on a person's life, in a way that acute pain typically does not. It can lead to loss of income, freedom, and family. There is evidence that individual factors can have a significant impact on how a person will respond to chronic pain. Often the originally injury has healed but the pain persists. The chronic pain is now behaving more like a disease.

Early studies of hypnotherapy to control chronic pain fared poorly, but much of this was related to the relatively poor quality of research available. With the course of time, the standards in research have improved significantly.

The area of chronic pain research and hypnosis that receives the most attention is headache. Overall, there is evidence that hypnosis can make a positive difference. However, so can autogenic training (which we use in our hypnotherapy training groups) and relaxation training. Nonetheless, it does not matter if hypnosis works as well as other interventions. The point is, there is evidence that it helps. Some people prefer relaxation training while others prefer to learn hypnosis. In this way, more interventions are made available to a larger number of people.

Research into other chronic pain conditions has found that hypnotherapy is more effective than doing nothing. However, it appears to be about as effective as relaxation training and autogenic training. Autogenic training was developed in Germany during the 1930s by psychiatrist Johannes Heinrich Schultz. His purpose was to find a universal method of inducing relaxation. As I tell patients who ask, if you are skilled at relaxation training or meditation, that is great. Now try adding some of the specific pain control methods I will show you later in this book and see if it works for you. Different people will find different methods to put their minds at ease. In this way, more interventions are made available to a larger number of people.

In 2014, a meta-analysis conducted by researcher Tomonorie Adachi and his colleagues at a Japanese university concluded that hypnotherapy does help to relieve chronic pain. A meta-analysis is created when a whole bunch of research is statistically melted down to represent one big experiment. This was an exciting finding, and my clinic was eager to check out the results of this paper. The researchers, we noted, focused on the question "Does hypnosis reduce pain?" Their answer was yes. However, they did not ask if hypnosis improves function or mood. It's an important question that deserves further research.

As a clinical physician, an academic, and a patient, I believe hypnosis can have some impact on pain. Some people will respond better than others. For most people, hypnosis is not likely to make their pain disappear. The treatment of chronic pain requires a team approach. A number of treatments might help, and hypnotherapy is one of them. It can help patients with chronic pain get some control of their pain. It might also help them reduce their use of potent, potentially addictive drugs. For me, hypnotherapy has been a very important tool and I am grateful that I learned how to use it. It might not be for everyone, but it is certainly worth a good clear examination before you reject it. The scientific literature seems to show us that there is some basis for the positive changes it seems to can bring to many patients.

Notes

1. The Stanford Hypnotic Susceptibility Scale and others like it raise several questions. Do they measure hypnotizability or waking suggestibility? Does a subject need to be formally hypnotized in order to be suggestible? It has also been suggested that this scale is not measuring hypnotizability but simply the desire to be hypnotized.

2. In state theories, hypnotic trance is associated with a physiologic change in brain function. State theories are represented by dissociation theories of hypnosis. Dissociation is a mental process in which there is a reduced connection between a person's thoughts, memories, feeling, physical sensations, actions, and even their sense of personal identity. There are a few variations, such as the theory of the hidden observer in hypnosis. Part of the subject's mind is aware of what is happening even if the hypnotized person is not. As a result, there is an "amnestic barrier" between the observer and the dissociated hypnotic subject.

    Then there is the theory by Woody and Bowers called the dissociated control theory of hypnosis

(DCT). In this model, when a highly hypnotizable person is hypnotized, their supervisory attentional system (SAS) or higher brain, frontal lobe functions become dissociated from the contention scheduling system (CS), which is considered a lower level system. This can be thought of as a behavioural system. So in effect, the frontal lobe becomes dissociated from a person's behavioural systems or "schemas." The hypnotist, through contextual cues and suggestions, can influence the CS or behaviours of the subject directly.

Finally, let us look at Gruzelier's neurophysiologic theory of hypnosis. This is another state theory. He described changes in brain function to explain hypnotic phenomena suggesting the more suggestible subjects had better executive functioning in the brain compared to less suggestible subjects. The more suggestible subjects were therefore more capable of using their attention in different ways. He went on to describe three levels of hypnosis. He postulated that the first part of hypnosis involved the left sided fronto-limbic system; during this time the subject is paying attention to the voice of the hypnotist. Next, there is a reduction in left fronto-limbic activity as the subject "lets go" and gives control to the hypnotist. The third stage of hypnosis sees an increase in right-sided tempero-posterior systems as the subject engages in passive imagery. It is thought that the frontal lobes "give up" and are functionally impaired in the hypnotic state.

3. There are problems with some of the research design and variation in how subjects are hypnotized. Mazzoni and colleagues put it well. In their 2013 paper they report on this controversy in the field of hypnosis. They look at whether hypnotic trance is a unique state of consciousness and, if it is, does it relate to suggestibility. They understand the problems with research to date on this subject. They conclude, as I have noted, that the data are equivocal "as to whether there is a causal relation between the changes in brain activity produced by hypnotic inductions and those produced by other suggestions. It also remains uncertain whether the changes in activation produced by hypnotic inductions reflect a uniquely hypnotic state as opposed to more mundane processes."

4. Oakley and his colleagues review the literature on experimental psychopathology as it relates to hypnosis. The objective is to find a "match" in imaging between the psychopathology in question and such pathology "induced" by hypnosis, similar to Halligan's case. However, not only can this model be used to understand conversion disorders, but it might also be used to understand delusional thinking, amnesia, migraine headache,

conversion disorder, somatic syndromes, chronic fatigue, irritable bowel syndrome, and certain painful conditions. It is important to recognize that a significant proportion of psychiatric illness is defined by subjective reports that are potentially amenable to hypnotic models. These clinicians suggest that hypnosis can be used to create "virtual patients" to help us understand certain illnesses and even disease. Of note, hypnotically induced pain activates those parts of the brain associated with pain perception, the same areas in patients with physically induced pain. Of interest, these areas of the brain do not activate when subjects are asked to imagine the pain.

5. In state theories of hypnosis, the subject is some-what passive in the process once they have been hypnotized. They give up control. In the cognitive behavioural theory of hypnosis, Spanos postulates that subjects use "role enactment." The subject transforms their imaginings, thoughts, and feeling into experiences and behaviours that fit their own idea of what makes a good hypnotic subject and they act accordingly. Hypnotic behaviour is really no different than non-hypnotic behaviour. How a person views hypnosis is a key determinant of the outcome of their hypnotic experience.

Finally, there are a number of theorists who do not see hypnosis as a state or non-state phenomena.

Rather, it is both. This is best explained by Kihlstrom: "It is clear what we should do, which is abandon the stance of either-or and adopt a new stance of both-and. This 'third way' in hypnosis research construes hypnosis simultaneously as both a state of (sometimes) profound cognitive change, involving basic mechanisms of cognition and consciousness, and as a social interaction, in which hypnotist and *subject come together for a specific purpose within a wider socio-cultural context*."

8

The Hypnotherapy for Pain Control Program

As a pain specialist, I am concerned about the use of opioid therapy and the poor outcomes I see from this treatment. Hypnotherapy provides a potentially safe alternative. I'd taught hypnotherapy to many patients for the past 30 years, one at a time, here and there. But in 2013, I decided to teach it to other people in a more organized way. I set up a group program, with people who had chronic pain.

This first group had eight people in it from all walks of life. There was Bill, who has been a volunteer in my group programs for the past eight years. He is one tough-looking biker dude, but he is the kindest of gentlemen. He worked as a pipe fitter. He had been hurt about 25 years before and no one would help him. I think he intimidated health care providers without meaning to—their loss. We got together in 2009 and I got him into my pain program. He did amazingly well. Right after he entered the program, he had a heart attack and because of the program, he managed that too. When I started the hypnotherapy group he was first in line. There was Susan who was struggling as a rehabilitation therapist. She was working full-time but because of injuries she had suffered in a car accident, she was at very high risk of leaving her job. She was struggling every day. There was Peter. Peter is an old patient of mine. He used to be an athletic fellow who would run 10 kilometres without thinking twice about it. Then he developed rheumatoid arthritis and was now on high doses of opioids. He wanted to get off them. He hated how they made him feel, but he didn't know what else to do with the pain. I was honoured to have Graham in the group. He was over 80 and had helped to build something that the world had never seen before. I can't tell you what it was or you would know who he is right away, but because of his work, he had met the Queen of England. William was an unemployed steel worker who spent most of his day doing nothing and feeling very badly about himself. Mary had horrible, unrelenting headaches. She used to work as an accountant, but now could do nothing. Muriel was a map maker. She had suffered an injury to her right arm that made it difficult to work—in fact, she had not worked in years. She had been in my pain program and had made great gains. She was working part-time but was struggling and was looking for something to control the pain. Finally there was Adrianne. I had taught her self-hypnosis skills many years before. She had used them with good success, until more recently, when she had been diagnosed with lupus and felt overwhelmed. She wanted a booster course. This was our first group. Pain does not pick and choose, it can strike anyone, rich, poor, tall or short. Like birth, death, and taxes, it knows no strangers.

I was very clear with each patient who entered my program. The goal of the program was to teach them how to use hypnotherapy to control their pain. I was not going to be the hypnotherapist who would control each session, do something to them, and lessen their pain. They would have to listen, ask questions, and practise, practise, and then practise some more. If they were not prepared to commit to practising there was no point in them coming into my program. They would not succeed. I also explained, as you now know, that some people learn hypnosis very easily while others, like me, don't. However, at the end of the day it does not make a difference. If you're willing to commit to practising, you'll get it. I did. It took me a year, but I got it and I've benefited ever since.

The program runs in the same facility—a local church—I use for my pain group program that has been running for almost twenty years. That first day is always exciting and scary for people. Imagine going into a room with seven other people you've never met and you're going to learn something a bit weird and a bit different—hypnosis. The only thing you might know about it is from that time when your friend had a hypnotist come to a Christmas party two years ago. He had your friend convinced he was in love with the first person he saw after he opened his eyes from the trance. Nothing bad happened but it was bizarre. How can that sort of thing help with pain?

It takes about three sessions before people become comfortable with one another. Then things become more settled. On that first day I introduce them to my co-therapist, Gilda, who is of course my wife and has worked in the field of pain longer than I have. I have Gilda as a co-therapist for two reasons. First, I think it is important for people to hear a different voice than mine and I want to have both genders present. The second reason is it's a great excuse for us to work together.

I also introduce everyone to my volunteer, Peter. Peter is the fellow I described to you. He is the long-distance runner with rheumatoid arthritis, trying to get off opioids. When I first met Peter, he was taking a lot of morphine. I taught him self-hypnosis, one on one, in my clinic. He took to it immediately. He could put himself into a very deep trance and demonstrate deep trance phenomena. More important, when he did self-hypnosis, his pain went from an 8 to 9 out of 10 to zero. That's right, zero. He was a phenomenon. He reduced his morphine. Unfortunately his disease got worse and his morphine dose had increased by the time he came to the group. I have used him as a volunteer in every group I have run to date to show people the best possible outcome, while I represent the other end of that scale.

Similar to most hospital-based treatment programs, we do "outcome" research. The purpose of this research is to make sure that what we do has some clinical value. On day one, patients complete a research package. They are given it again at the end of the program and we use these data to determine if anything has changed. In the package is the Stanford Hypnotic Suggestibility Scale. Although this scale has been criticized, it is the best of what we have to measure a person's ability to be hypnotized. The rest of the package measures things like pain, function, and the presence of any psychiatric problems.

I have run six group programs—which is not really enough yet to make any comment from the research data. What I can tell you from my observations, however, is that the vast majority of patients who come benefit. As in any treatment, some do not benefit as much as the treating physician would like, but I think it is because these patients do not practise enough. How do I know these things? Because I see these people in follow-up and they tell me what is happening for them. It might not be as potent as good research, but it does tell me that people who make the effort do learn the skill and start to take some control of their pain. A few reduce their reliance on medications like opioids. That is a huge improvement and alone is worth the price of admission.

The vast majority of the patients who attend the program have already been through my 15-week-long multidisciplinary pain program. They understand that they have to figure out how they're going to have a life—in spite of their pain. In the 15-week program, I do one session on hypnotherapy to introduce patients to the concept, so the people who are in the hypnotherapy program have some understanding of what the program is about. In truth a person has to be "well enough" to do the program. If they are very depressed, they wouldn't have the ability to concentrate or practise to learn the skill successfully.

I use a method of hypnosis based on the work of Milton Erickson, who saw hypnosis as a way of taking advantage of the natural processes of human beings. We might not be aware of it, but we are going in and out of trances all the time. It really doesn't have to be forced on anyone. It works better to invite patients to enter into a trance state that they have experienced before without thinking about it. This method simply gets people to do what they have already been doing, without realizing it.

On Day One, I do something a little bit odd. I do some stage hypnosis. I do this demonstration to make it clear to the patients that what they are about to do is not stage hypnosis, usually the only kind of hypnosis they know about. I already know that Paul is a great subject so I don't have to do any selection exercises. I usually do some type of dramatic induction. We start with Paul and me standing. I usually dramatically touch him on his forehead, push back, and say, "Sleep." He slumps back into his chair in a trance. I deepen the trance and then give him a suggestion. The one I usually do is have him forget the number 6 in a counting sequence. I go through the process with him and then "wake" him up from the trance. I have him count. Nine times out of ten he does forget 6. The odd time he stumbles over it and then remembers it. I usually do the stage act fairly quickly—if only to show people that stage hypnosis is for entertainment. It's not clinical hypnosis, which in our case is meant to help people lessen the feeling of pain. That is the last time we speak about it.

Day One is not over yet. On this first day, we give patients their first peek at the basis of hypnosis, a skill critical to learning hypnotic induction. This important skill is something we all do every day. What is it? Breathing. That's right: simple breathing. The only problem is most of us are panting and shallow-breathing throughout the day. It is rare for most people to fill their lungs when they breathe—and there is nothing wrong with this. It will not harm you. But in order to learn how to put yourself into a trance, you must learn to control your breathing before you can do anything else.

We tell people to practise these skills in a comfortable environment, but not lying down. The goal is to be able to use these skills anywhere. If you start by learning how to do them lying down, you'll have a much longer way to go to learn how to use them standing up. Sit comfortably in a chair and start from there. This is where we show people "square breathing" techniques. This skill is simple on the surface but takes a bit of time to master. I'll describe these breathing techniques in some detail in the next chapter.

I might also show patients what is sometimes referred to as "mindful movement." These are movements that for some people increase the impact of the breathing technique. For me, that's all it is, a way to improve the ability to breathe properly and relax—I'm not teaching people how to transcend this life. I'm just trying to show patients a technique that might help them focus better on themselves and help to shut out the noise of the world for a little while. It might improve their capacity to learn to breathe properly and relax.

Week Two begins with Gilda doing an autogenic exercise, which means self-generated, training session. It's another form of hypnosis, meditation, and relaxation. The goal of Johannes Schultz, who had studied hypnosis and other methods for calming an individual, was to develop a method whereby a patient could calm themselves and not rely on a therapist. Autogenics typically works from a script that is read through and it is by concentrating on the words and language of the script that a person is helped to relax. After the first autogenic script, patients learn their very first induction. Hypnotic induction is the business of putting a person into the right state so that they can go into a different state of mind, a hypnotic trance.

Next is the first hypnotic induction. This method was developed by me specifically as a simple, mobile method. It begins by simply staring at your hand. The next part is a deepening exercise to make people have either a deeper trance or simply to become even more relaxed. I end this session by bringing patients to a relaxing scene that they can remember and use again when they practise. The rest of this session is spent practising what has been taught. I don't teach pain control methods until we are about halfway through the program. Patients first have to learn how to settle and relax themselves, understand self-hypnosis, and develop the ability to do it, before they can their learn to control pain.

In Weeks Three and Four, people are introduced to other induction methods, of which there are many. I gradually make each method a bit more complicated than the one before. I also try to show people that they can use a variety of senses to get there. The most common sense used in hypnosis is sight, but I teach an induction based on taste and one based on sound. Just to be clear, there is no evidence that a more complicated induction will work better than a simple one. In fact, there is no significant research of any kind showing that one type of hypnosis is dramatically better than another—I just prefer elements of the Ericksonian methods. So if the only thing you learn is the simplest method, that's great. Some people prefer more razzle-dazzle to become engaged in the process of learning. There really is something for everyone if you are willing to look.

Week Five is special. I now introduce patients to pain control. There is a fairly long list of pain control methods associated with hypnosis. Here are some of them.

- Once a person is in a trance and relaxed, I teach them to transfer that sense of relaxation to the pain itself. Sounds strange. But it works. I have them relax the muscles and bone and nerves around the painful area. If they can, actually "relax the pain." Simple idea, but one that works well.

- Another simple method is to have the patient "forget" the pain. This is really based on a phenomenon called dissociation, in which a person can make a part of themselves become less important. In dissociation, a person in a trance can make a part of themselves seem more distant, almost not attached. If you do this to a painful area, the pain can reduce.

- A very interesting method is inducing analgesia to the area of pain. One of the inductions I teach is actually an analgesic induction, and if it's successful, the area of analgesia can spread. I actually start doing this in a non-painful area, inducing a sense of numbness like you get with a local anaesthetic. I then have the patient transfer this feeling to the painful area. When it works, it is quite shocking. One patient actually smelled lidocaine when they did this and they got excellent results!

- Another method that I use a lot is "fixing" the pain. I have the patient imagine what they think is causing the pain, imagine what is broken. Because I know anatomy and pathology, I know exactly why

I have the pain and I can imagine it very clearly. Someone else might imagine their pain coming from a broken circuit board while another person might see it more like a broken wood structure. It does not make a difference. Once you have an image of what is broken, try to fix it in your mind's eye. When this works, it is quite powerful.

- The colour potpourri and the change of count are classic and simple methods of pain control in hypnosis. In colour potpourri, the person imagines the pain as a colour. They then imagine its opposite colour. I don't expect patients to know colour theory—they don't have to know the real opposite colour. Whatever colour they think is the opposite will do just fine. They then allow the opposite colour to mix into the painful colour until the healthy colour takes over the whole image. The change in count is a separate method but I often attach it to the colour potpourri. These are my two favourite methods of pain control. In the change of count, the patient is asked to imagine their pain as a number. Choosing numbers in the range of 1 to 10 is usually easiest. Once the person has the number, I ask them to "morph" the number and twist it and change it so that it reduces by one and as it does to allow the pain to reduce as well. The trick is to not simply twist the number in your mind. The pain must follow along. Slowly, slowly. If a person succeeds, they can try doing it again. (There's more about these methods in the last chapter.)

From Week Five a new format is used in each session. It starts with autogenics followed by a new induction, and finally a method of pain control is added. This format goes on through to Week Nine.

Finally we get to Week Ten. This is the final group, and it's different than the rest. In this group every participant brings in an induction that they have developed based on the principles that have been taught in the group. Then they have to teach it to the rest of us. If a person can do that, I know they understand the principles of self-hypnosis and they will develop the necessary skill to control their pain.

It's inspiring to hear my own patients tell the group what hypnosis has done to alleviate their pain. Take Bill, the biker. He took the hypnotherapy course very seriously and practised every day. Then, after about four months, he told me that he got it. Now he uses this method just about every day. He is able to use less medication and is doing amazingly well. If you ask him, he will tell you that it changed his life.

The Myths of Hypnosis

The Internet is filled with page after page of references to myths in hypnosis. No matter what anyone says on the Internet about hypnosis, the truth is no one has done any research on these myths. I know this for a fact because my clinic actually did check to see if there was any research data to support or refute the myths of hypnosis. However, based on my clinical experience, I have found that the information on the Internet simply reflects the fears that the general public have about the hypnotic process. This is borne out of believing clinical hypnosis is the same as stage hypnosis. As we have seen, that is clearly not the case. These are the most common myths:

- People in hypnosis can lose complete control.

- People may not be able to come out of hypnosis.

- Hypnosis affects only weak-willed or gullible people.

- Hypnosis reliably enhances the accuracy of memory.

- Hypnosis enables people to re-experience a past life.

- Hypnosis depends primarily on the skill of the hypnotist.

There are also some common questions about hypnosis:

Is hypnosis sleep?

No, hypnosis is not sleep although when the name hypnosis was developed it was thought that the process was a form of sleep. We now know this is not the case and the name hypnosis (Greek for "to put to sleep") is a misnomer.

Can anyone be hypnotized?

We know that it is difficult for some people to be hypnotized, like me. However, if you work hard enough even if you have difficulty being hypnotized, eventually you will get it.

Can I be forced to do something I don't want to do?

The idea that a hypnotist can make you do things you don't want to do is a significant fear for many people. If you know the history of hypnosis, you know there are some very famous cases where people have used hypnosis as an excuse for murder. They claim that they had no control and were under the power of the hypnotist. Fortunately, these claims are extremely infrequent. They also don't seem to hold up in court. I'm quite good at doing hypnotic inductions and I have yet to make anyone do anything they do not want to do. I can assure you that in doing self-hypnosis, you will not have to worry about doing anything you don't want to do.

Will I be in a hypnotic trance forever?

Perhaps the most common fear is that somehow a person will not come out of a hypnotic trance. I assure you, when that person gets hungry enough, they will come out of the trance.

Although no formal research has been done on the subject of the myths of hypnosis, in my clinical experience and based on my clinic's review of the literature, hypnosis will not cause you harm and can only do you some good. Give it a try.

9

Outside In:
How to Hypnotize
Yourself for Pain
Relief

I n this chapter I will show you how to hypnotise yourself, using the traditional style of hypnosis. In the clinical setting, I start by building a rapport with the patient. The next step is to analyze the patient's problems and come up with a treatment plan that might include hypnotherapy. If hypnotherapy is used, we start with the induction. Remember, you're not actually being "induced" to do something. Rather, you're being invited. My job is to create an atmosphere in which you choose to go into a trance state. The following pages show several inductions. If you're successful, this will lead to a state called absorption. Absorption means exactly what it says. You become absorbed by something. In the case of hypnosis you are initially absorbed by the induction, the process of being hypnotized. Absorption is not an unusual state and people go through it all the time.

A good example of absorption occurs when you watch a long movie and forget about everything around you. You become absorbed by the film. This is how hypnosis begins. You start by doing an induction and if you are doing it correctly you forget about what is going on around you.

If you keep at it and practise, eventually you will enter the next stage, called dissociation. In dissociation, you become more clearly detached from the world around you. If dissociation becomes even deeper, you become detached from physical experiences like pain. It is a detachment from reality, not a loss of reality. I don't carry the induction process further than this. Once a patient learns to dissociate, they can do an action of some type. It might be pain control or relaxation. Finally there is the ending of the session.

Of course, there's a difference between reading the words here and being in a clinical session with me. A book lacks the dynamic of human contact. You have to approach things a bit differently. Start with the simplest breathing exercises. Read through them again. Pick one and practise it. If you are not sure about it, read it again and practise again. Practise repeatedly until you're confident that you've got it. Then go on to the next induction, slowly working your away along.

An iPad app follows the content of this chapter. The app contains my work and the work of my staff. You can find it at http://hypnotherapyforpaincontrol.com.

When I teach self-hypnosis I always start with the breathing. Most of us are shallow-breathing, at relatively high speed all day. If you can get control of your breathing, you will automatically calm down. Even if you don't learn specific pain control methods, calming down and relaxing will automatically reduce your pain.

At the start of every session in our group program, my co-therapist, Gilda, gets people ready to go to the next stage. She begins with breathing. We usually use box breathing (described below), but other methods, which I will also describe, work just as well. She then does an auto-genic form of trance induction. One of the basic principles of autogenics is repetition. For example, a statement like "Relax my arm" will be repeated multiple times. I like to expand the statement each time: "Relax my arm and feel the muscles become less tense. Relax my arm and feel each finger lose tension and simply curl a bit" and so on.

Here's another example: You might say to yourself, "My right arm feels heavy." You repeat this to yourself four to six times, and each time you might expand the statement: "My right arm feels heavy like it's asleep. It's so heavy that it feels like the muscles have gone to sleep" and so on.

Before we begin looking at hypnotic induction, though, you must learn how to breathe again. Breathing to relax is critical in this process. For some people, this alone reduces their pain.

Breathing Techniques

Let's begin. First, get comfortable in a chair. Try to wear comfortable clothing when you do this. Do not do this lying down or it will be more difficult for you to learn how to do this when you are standing up and that's where you want to be at the end of your training. Take a minute to just pay attention to how you're breathing right now. Is it shallow? Is it fast? You can even count the number of breaths you're taking in a minute. This helps you understand what you're doing. Now let's try to modify your breathing for the better.

Box Breathing

One of the simplest methods of preparing for an induction is called box breathing. Either imagine or draw a box on a piece of paper. I draw a rectangle that is wider than it is tall—you will see why. Now, pattern your breathing using the box outline as a guide. As you breathe in, follow the top of the box. Hold your breath briefly as you go down the first side of the box. Breathe out while your eye travels along the second long side of the box, and finally hold again on the last short side of the box. Now keep the pattern up. Some people find it easier at first to use a finger and follow the box they have drawn as they breathe. Take your time with this. Make sure you've got it. Now, slow your breathing down. Not a lot. Just a little bit. You do this by simply changing the rhythm of how you visualize the box. It's even easier if you use your finger. Now you see why I draw a rectangle. When you breathe, inhalation and exhalation are longer than the pauses between each act. Keep this up. Now lengthen the arm of each part of your box/

rectangle. So your inhalation is a bit longer, you hold it longer, your exhalation is longer, and you hold it longer. Take your time with this. As you master this method, start slowing it down more and more. Perhaps you can get your breathing down by 10 percent to start. Eventually maybe even 30 percent. Slow it up. Practise this very simple exercise. It doesn't seem like much, but it is very important—if you don't control your breathing, you might as well forget about doing the rest. Don't go on to doing an induction until you get this down by practising every day.

Bumble Bee Breathing or Bhramari Pranayama

This form of breathing comes from yoga. (Bhramari is named after the Indian black bee and pranayama refers to control of breath.) I am not teaching you yoga, simply an interesting breathing technique. This way you have two options. In classic bumble bee breathing, you start with your fingers in your ears, pushing on the cartilage of the ear between your cheek and ear. You don't have to do this to get the effect I'm interested in, but many people find it makes the method work better. At some point, once you are in a relaxed state, I suggest you remove your fingers from you ears.

Either way, start in a comfortable sitting position with your fingers in your ears or not. In classic yoga, you would be in a Padmasana or Lotus type position. However, we're doing hypnosis, not classic yoga. Start breathing in through both nostrils. Slowly. Now, when you breathe out, make a humming sound. That's the bee. You might want to start with a 3-second inhalation and 4- to 5-second exhalation. Keep it up. Focus on the sound you're making. Try to forget everything else except that sound. Keep it up but now try a 4-second inhalation and a 5- to 6-second exhalation. When I do this, I use my fingers to count the seconds so I don't have to look at a watch, which screws up my concentration. I'm focusing on the wrong thing. Focus on your breathing. Stretch it out. See how long you can take for each stage of this process. You might want to keep your inhalation at 5 seconds but just extend the exhalation. See if you can push that up to 10. With practice maybe you can get to 6 seconds of inhalation and 12 seconds of exhalation. Now go silent. Maintain the breathing pattern but without the sound. Fun stuff. If you just learn how to breathe right, you can make your pain less. You don't have to do anything more if you don't want to.

Movement

There is a tradition of movements associated with breathing. For some people, these movements can deepen the relaxed feeling they get. Let me tell you about a few of them. These are called "mindful movements." The simplest one involves raising your arms above your head as you inhale, and as you exhale, lowering your arms to your sides. If that's uncomfortable, lower them to your front. It's the movement that's the point. You can even stretch your hands and fingers when you get to the top of the arc and then relax everything as you exhale and move your arms down. If one arm hurts, just do the movement with the arm that doesn't.

Do the same movement but now interlock your fingers at the top of the arc, rotate your hands so they face upwards and push up. Stretch and stretch. Now, exhale, let your arms come down, and relax.

Here is one more. Place your fingertips together (not clasped) with your hands resting on your lap. As you inhale, bring your hands up to about the level of your chin. When you exhale take your hands down into your lap. You can do a more complex version of this: as you bring your hands up to your chin, rotate your hands, fingertips still touching, so that the palms are touching your chin. It's as if you're resting your head in the cup created by your interlocked fingers.

Mindful movements can get quite complicated and can include legs and feet. However, I'm not trying to teach you this technique. I would prefer you do the breathing exercises seated for now since that is the position we will work from for doing hypnosis. I'm describing the option of adding a bit of movement to the breathing if it makes it easier for you.

The most important next step is to practise, practise, practise until this becomes second nature.

Now, let's put breathing and autogenics together.

First, get into a comfortable seated position. Begin with the breathing that you now know how to do. Set the tone. Slow your breathing down. Now do a body scan. Notice where you feel relaxed and where you feel tense. Let yourself feel calm inside. If you want to, close your eyes. Now, paying attention to your right arm, let it feel warm. Perhaps the warmth starts in a small area on your hand or shoulder. Repeat the idea to yourself three to six times, expanding the suggestion. Say you are feeling the warmth on your baby finger. Try feeling it, finger by finger, until all your fingers feel warm. Be creative: Your arm, forearm, and hand are now completely warm and very relaxed. Now pay attention to your left arm. See if you can make the left arm feel exactly like your right arm. This is a common way to transfer feeling from one area of the body to another. Let your left arm, forearm, and hand become warm and relaxed. Once again, repeat multiple times, expanding the feeling. Now your right and left arms, forearms, and hands are relaxed and warm.

Expand the warmth from your arms into your chest. Let it flow like water into your chest; as the area gets warmer, the muscles relax. Repeat several times, expanding the idea. Your chest is now as warm and relaxed as your upper limbs. Let the warmth continue to spread down to your stomach. Feel your stomach become warmer and warmer and the muscles relax more and more. You now know the routine. Expand the idea. Repeat it. Let the warmth wrap around to your lower back, spreading upward to your upper back.

Your entire back, from top to bottom is warm and relaxed. Pay attention to your right leg. Begin at the top and allow your thigh to heat up and become warm. Feel the heat and as the heat increases, the muscles become more relaxed. (Expand.) Allow the feeling to flow down to your leg and calf. Again, allow this area to become warmer and warmer and as it does, allow the muscles to relax, to simply let go. Now let the heat move into your feet. Feel it spread as the small muscles relax. Allow the entire lower limb to warm up and relax. As you did before, let these muscles also heat up. Become warmer and warmer. As they warm up the tension releases and the muscles relax. Now, like you did with your arms, extend the feeling from the right side to the left. Allow your left leg, calf, and foot to warm up and become comfortably hot. As the area heats up, the muscles become relaxed, less tense.

Moving back up to your arms, let the warmth that is there, on both sides, flow up into your neck from each side. Your neck does not have to become limp, but it can become very relaxed. Warmer and warmer, more relaxed. As before, use the same methods to relax this area. From the neck, allow the heat to move up to your face. Take your time. Let it move into every nook and cranny of your face. Bit by bit. Around your chin, mouth, nose, eyes, and ears. Let the heat twist around to the back of your head until your entire head is warm. (Repeat and expand.)

Now your entire body and head should feel warm and relaxed.

Feel the relaxation in your entire body and a pleasant feeling of warmth and heaviness. Take a few moments now to just relax. Relax for a few moments longer, enjoying the feelings of calm and warmth.

When you are ready to finish this autogenic exercise, tell yourself that when you return to being fully alert, you do not have to become tense: "I can still stay relaxed." Start by breathing deeply. Move your arms and legs, hands and feet. Stretch. Allow your muscles to feel firm without being tense. Let your eyes open. Take a moment and breathe in and out. You are ready to go to the next stage.

When I am teaching hypnosis, I begin each session with a brief autogenic exercise to get everyone set and in the right state of mind. If you did this exercise, you have just introduced yourself to a form of hypnotic induction.

Your First Formal Hypnotic Inductions
Simple Induction

There is no evidence that a complicated method of induction works better than a simple one so I'm going to describe the simplest possible method of induction. It's based more on what you say to yourself than anything else and contains all the basic principles of self-hypnosis: breathing (plus or minus autogenics), deepening, relaxation and return. I will introduce you to pain control a bit later. First you have to master the induction.

Start with your breathing. You can include an autogenic element if you like. The breathing should be straightforward for you, using the method you prefer. Take your time. Get a good rhythm to your breathing and then slow it down by at least 20 percent. Nice and slow.

Now, find a spot that is easy for you to look at for a long time. Make sure it's something completely inanimate. This might sound like a strange rule but I always include it because years ago a patient told me they had a lot of trouble with this beginning part. Why? They had picked a spot on their dog. Make sure that the spot you pick cannot move! Stare at the spot and let your eyes slowly relax.

Now, paying attention to your breathing, take one deep breath, in and out. Just like box breathing. Now take another. Do this five times. With each breath out, say to yourself, "Relax, let the tension go in my body." You're still looking at that single spot. You might also pay a bit of attention to your eyes. Relax your eyes. They might even feel a bit heavy.

At the end of five breaths, take in a deep breath and hold to the count of five in your mind: "One, two, three, four, five." As you count, again let your body relax. You might be able to create an image of how that is happening. For me, when I do this, at the point of holding my breath I imagine a wave moving from the middle of my chest outward down my arms, legs, and up into my face, down to my hands and feet. As the wave moves, the tension inside of me reduces.

Now repeat the whole process again. Breathe in and out for five breaths. Remember to tell yourself to relax with each exhalation and at the end of the five breaths hold to the count of five. The mechanics are important but the self-talk is critical. You are continually telling yourself to relax and let tension go. Without that self-talk, you won't get anywhere. If you can create images of this, so much the better.

When your eyes have to close and your body feels very relaxed, you have most likely got yourself into a very light trance state. Now what do you do with it? We're not at the pain control stage yet—later I'll show you some pain control methods. For now, let's deepen your state of relaxation.

Deepening

In self-hypnosis, we start with some type of induction such as I've just described and then typically follow it with a method of deepening the trance. There are different ways of doing this. The classic method uses the idea of a stairwell as the image on which to focus. Once you have closed your eyes and you can feel yourself becoming even more relaxed, imagine a stairwell, with you standing at the top. People in a trance are usually able to imagine things very clearly. Give the image a lot of detail. You are in complete control of the image so if your stairs are rickety and feel unsafe, it's because you made them that way. If you do this, you will delay your progress. Who wants to go down a rickety set of stairs? So create a very safe, sturdy stairwell with railings so they're easy to go down. Create landings so you can rest. I make my stairwell circular because it works better for me. Once you have that image, give it colour and temperature. Make it pleasantly warm. Now start to walk down the stairs. Take your time. With each step down, tell yourself that you are becoming more relaxed. Step by step. If you don't feel more relaxed, don't keep walking down the steps. Move only as fast as your thinking will allow you to. If you want to take a break, create a landing and stop for a bit. Go back to your breathing. It is central to the process. Now return to the stairs, going down deeper and deeper until you feel ready to stop and once again create a landing and stop.

Relaxation

Now that you've deepened the state you're in, let's use it for the purpose of creating a very relaxed state. Let's use the state you're in to create a scenario that you can use for relaxation anytime you want. It's a good time to see how suggestible you really are. Once you've deepened your state, let the stairwell image fade away and replace it with a place you've been or would like to go to that you find very relaxing. Again, remember that you control the image so nothing is in it that you don't put there. If you have someone chasing you, it's because you put that character in your image. Get him out. Keep the image as relaxing as you can. Make sure you create the image with as much detail as you can. This includes sights, sounds, smells, temperatures, and even taste. Detail, detail, detail. Once you have the image, just let yourself relax there.

As you relax, give yourself a suggestion. Suggest to yourself that the next time you want to relax you're going to try a shortcut. First, you will remember the image you just created. When you're ready to get into this relaxed state, you will tell yourself, "I'm going to allow myself to go into a very relaxed state. I'm going back to the relaxing image I used the last time I was in a trance." You will then start your breathing. This time, you'll begin by slowing your breathing; once you've done that, count your breaths backwards from ten to one. With each breath, allow yourself to remember the last trance you created for yourself. Go deeper with each number counted. Once you get to one, you can decide if it feels deep enough. If it is, great. If not, do a deepening exercise, such as the one with the staircase image. Once it's deep enough, call up that relaxing image. Again, fill in the detail and spend some time there. Once again, when you finish, go through the process of placing the suggestion you just created in your mind.

When you do this for the first time on your own, it's possible that nothing will happen. That just means you need to practise the longer simple induction process again and try the suggestion again. If the suggestion works, great, but you should use it almost every day or it will fade out. Have fun with this one.

Return

It is now time to come back to the day-to-day world. I have one rule when I teach people self-hypnosis. If you want to stop, do not just "wake up." People get headaches when they do this. Nine times out of ten they have put themselves into a light trance and don't know it. When they jump up suddenly, they tend to pay for it with a headache. I can't explain why this happens but I have seen it over and over again for 30 years. So, if you have had enough or it's time to end, go through this very simple process. First, tell yourself that it's time to end. Remember where you are and remember to tell yourself that you can come back to this spot whenever you want to by starting with your breathing exercises again.

To come back from the deep state, plant the suggestion that you can return to the relaxed state by doing the breathing exercise. Now tell yourself that you're going to return to your day-to-day life. First, reverse your trip down the stairwell. Tell yourself to walk up the stairs, and with each step up you become progressively more alert and more aware. You don't have to rush this. Take your time. Step by step. The banter is important so continue to watch yourself walk up the steps, making sure you don't break into a run; don't allow yourself to become tense in the process. More alert, more aware, but still relaxed. Once you get to the top of the stairs, tell yourself that you're going to take 10 deep breaths and that at the fifth breath, your eyes will open. With every breath in, you become progressively more aware of the environment around you. Breathe in once. Again tell yourself to become a bit more alert. Feel the chair underneath you. Hear the sounds in the room.

Breathe in again. This is breath two. Repeat the same ideas. Repeat slowly for five breaths. At the fifth breath, your eyes should open. Start taking in what you see as you continue to breathe. Tell yourself that you can maintain a sense of relaxation even though you're coming out of a trance. You don't have to be tense to be awake. Become more aware of your environment until you reach ten. You are now back.

Remember the basic structure of each session: breathing, induction, deepening, and relaxation. I will add pain control a bit later once you have mastered the hypnotic induction. Let's try another induction.

Basic Induction: "The Wrinkles of Your Hand"

Once you have mastery of your breathing, you're ready to move on to learning how to do a basic hypnotic induction. I developed this method because it is simple and straightforward. You don't need any special equipment. You always have the equipment with you. This method is something I developed for a film that was made of me doing hypnotherapy on a patient. The goal was to design something that was easy to do and easy to teach.

Sitting comfortably, start by using one of your breathing methods. Begin this method with your eyes open. I'll let you know when you can close them if you want to. Now place one of your hands on top of the other, palms up.

Bring your palms close to your face so you can see the lines on your hands very clearly. Keep breathing. If you're using Brahmari breathing (bumble bee breathing), go from making the sound to silence. Look at some point on the palm of your hand. Find a line or area that captures your interest and look at that one area only while maintaining your breathing. You are using a method of hypnotic induction called eye fixation. It's just like the classic image of the hypnotist with the watch going back and forth, but without the watch. Breathe and focus on the area of your hand. Now, as you breathe in, imagine that you're bringing in fresh, healing air that fills your body. It completely fills you up and as the breath moves in, you can feel yourself feeling a bit better. As you go into exhalation, imagine you're expelling anything negative inside of you. As you do this, keep your eyes open. Do not close them yet. Breathing in and out, inhale a positive feeling and exhale a negative one. You might even be able to put an image to this movement, perhaps imagining that as you exhale you're pushing your pain out of your body. This is your first pain control technique. Keep this process up. It never works to rush it. You are now the hypnotherapist. You are telling yourself what to do. Breathe in and out slowly. Inhale a positive feeling and exhale negative feelings or even pain. As you say this banter to yourself, see if you can do it to the rhythm of your breathing. If you can't imagine what I'm suggesting, don't rush ahead. Stick with it. Practise again and again until you can get a feel for what I'm suggesting. Eventually you might notice that your eyes are fluttering or they feel very heavy. This can be the indication of the start of a light trance. Do not rush to close your eyes just yet. Keep up the process. In and out, inhale the positive and exhale the negative. Slow and rhythmic breathing. Perhaps your eyes are watering a bit. Don't worry. This is all expected. It's normal. You might start to notice that your eyes are hard to keep open. Resist the desire to close them if you can. Just continue to breathe, and imagine inhaling something positive and exhaling the negative feelings in your body. Look closely at your hand. Notice the lines, the swirls, the minute details. When you reach a point where you simply cannot keep your eyes open, let them close. Now repeat to yourself, "Relax, relax, relax." Pay attention to your breathing.

This might seem very simple, but some people have trouble letting themselves go into a light trance. Don't worry about it. Be honest with yourself. Keep practising. Don't go on to a new trance method until you master this one. It does not get much simpler.

Once you have allowed yourself to go into a light trance, it's time to use another method of deepening the effect.

Deepening

I have already shown you the stairwell method. It's a classic, but it's not the one I tend to use. I use the image of an elevator. Imagine an elevator at the top of an endlessly tall building. Create the image of the inside of the elevator.

Give it as much detail as you can. Give it sounds and smells. If you can feel the cold walls of the elevator, that's great. Perhaps your elevator is warm. Detail, detail, detail. Now, in your mind's eye, go into the elevator on the top floor. Close the doors. In front of you is an endlessly large panel of buttons that will take you down in the elevator. Pick a floor and push the button. As the elevator moves down, allow yourself to feel a sense of deepening. As the elevator continues down, allow yourself to feel progressively more relaxed and less tense. Let yourself become more relaxed floor by floor. Do not go too fast. Allow the elevator to move to the next floor only when you feel more relaxed. Bit by bit, and floor by floor, you are becoming more relaxed. When you feel ready, allow the elevator to come to a stop.

Relax

In the previous induction I gave you a method to deepen relaxation by creating an image. Do that again here. Get good at it. It's a very good way to relax yourself.

Return

Once again, when you're ready it's time to return to the neutral start. You already did this before. Do the same thing except instead of going up a flight of stairs, you're going to recreate the image of the elevator. You're going to take the elevator up, floor by floor. With each floor up, you become progressively more alert and more aware of your environment. Just like before. Take your time. Feel the movement upward and feel yourself becoming more alert with each floor. Once you get to the top, allow the elevator to disappear. Like before, count forward from one to ten and allow yourself to become more alert with each breath in until you are back to the start. Remember, you can come out of a trance without becoming more tense.

You now have two very simple trance induction methods, plus two methods of deepening, and a method for deepening relaxation. You have a method for a post-hypnotic suggestion and a method for getting back to neutral. Pretty good. Next I'm going to tell you about my favourite method of induction, which I have taught for over 20 years. I have used this method on patients who were certain they could never learn how to do this. This is the method I used when I first learned hypnosis and when I finally got it. Given that I have shown you two methods of deepening, I won't show you that again. I will just tell you when to do it. The same is true of how to reverse the trance. You already know how to do that too.

Eyelid Induction

If you learn no other induction, learn this one. You already have a feel for the structure of an induction and the importance of the internal banter. The banter is important in every induction you do. Let's get started.

Begin with breathing. Then find a spot to look at. Make sure when you do this that you're physically as comfortable as you can be. Remember, don't do this lying down. Just look at that spot. In this induction, the focus is on your eyes. Pay attention to your eyes. Tell yourself:

"I am going to count backwards from 10 to 1. At 5 my eyes will close." How do I know this will happen? Simple: you will not say five to yourself until your eyes are ready to close. This means if you're not ready the first time you try this induction, so be it. Maybe the next time or perhaps the 20th time. Stick with it and you'll get there, but don't force it or pretend. If you're not ready to let go, you simply aren't and forcing it won't improve anything. You will also say: "As I count backwards, I will pay attention to how heavy my eyelids feel. Ten means I am completely alert while 9 means my eyes are a bit heavier. By 5 my eyes will feel so heavy I cannot keep them open." Now begin.

Ten. Give it a bit of time and you'll start to notice that your eyes feel a bit heavy. It's hard to keep your eyes focused perhaps. Once you're clear in your mind that you're not completely alert, as you were at the start, say "Nine" to yourself. Continue in the same way, paying attention to your eyes. "My eyes are starting to water a bit perhaps. They feel heavy and when I try to keep them open it's a bit more difficult." When there's a clear difference, say "Eight." Continue in this way until you get to six. The jump between six and five is significant. Do not say "Five" to yourself until your eyes feel so heavy, you have no choice but to close them. Then say "Five" and let your eyes close. From five to one, you are going to count backwards. Each number lets you feel progressively more relaxed. Keep your breathing rhythmic. Five, more relaxed and less tense; four, breathing is rhythmic and you can feel the tension melting away. Perhaps you can create an image. I have the image of water flowing out of my body and with it all the tension in it. Three, two, and one. Each number down, continue the banter. Now use a deepening method.

I have already shown you two deepening methods but the number of methods is as endless as your imagination. I scuba dive, so I've used the image of going underwater to deepen my trance. I have also used sky diving. You get the idea. Here is where you can be creative once you get some confidence in the process.

Pain Control

Previously we have gone from deepening to relaxation. This time we are going to move to pain control. This is a classic method of pain control called the colour potpourri, which I briefly described earlier. I mix it with another method, which I call morphing. This way you get two methods at one time. Let's begin.

Before you start this, do one of the hypnotic inductions and deepen it. Now, instead of going to a relaxing place, do a pain control method like this one. Imagine in your mind's eye your pain as a colour. It can be any colour you like. There is no right or wrong about this. Some people think of their pain as hot so they might think of red. Others feel their pain as cold so they think of blue. You might have a completely different colour. Whatever it is, give your pain a colour and a clear image in your mind in that colour. Now, imagine the opposite colour. I am not asking you to be colour theorists. Colours do have an opposite and when they are mixed they create a grey. That's not what I'm after here. The opposite colour is whatever you decide it is. What colour would you see if you were pain free? That's the colour I'm after. Once you have the opposite colour, great. Now allow this opposite colour to slowly leak into the colour image you have of your pain. Let the colours mix. Perhaps when they mix, you get a grey or perhaps the colours disappear. Make sure that when the colours mix they nullify one another in some way that is meaningful to you. Keep mixing in more and more of the opposite colour. Do not go faster, however, than you actually feel. If your pain is not reducing, don't keep mixing. Let the pain reduction catch up to your image and then continue along. When you hit a point where there is no more change in pain, stop. That's fine.

Now, with the colours in mind, give your pain a number. It's easier to do this out of 10. Again, there is no right or wrong. Once you have a number, imagine it in your mind very clearly. Now slowly bend the shape of the number, in your mind's eye, until you go down by one number. If you started at 7, you should now be at 6. Take your time with this. Don't change the number again, until you feel a change in your pain. Continue with this until you are no longer getting any change in your pain.

Fractionation

I would not be teaching you self-hypnosis properly if I didn't introduce you to what is called fractionation. It is used to describe a method of going into a trance, coming out, and going right back in again, perhaps three or even four times. You will see that this process deepens a trance relatively quickly.

Here is a very simple induction ideal for fractionation. Breathe in and out slowly five times; now hold your breath for five seconds. That is it. Repeat this and as you do, tell yourself to relax. With each breath in, relax. As you hold your breath, allow the tension in your body to reduce. Repeat this over and over until you feel relaxed. Now use a deepening method. Once you feel you are in a deep enough trance, bring yourself out of it and repeat it immediately. If you prefer, you can use one of the methods I've described above instead of this new one. Repeat the process three or four times. Now try a pain control method you have learned and see if it is more or less effective.

Pain Control Method

Remember, before you do any of the pain control methods you must be able to easily do a hypnotic induction and deepen it. You know you are doing it right if you can get yourself into a very relaxed state. I refer to this pain control method as "the mechanism." In your mind's eye, imagine the mechanism that is creating your pain. Use what you know. For example, if you're a carpenter, your image might be made out of wood with some areas that are rotten. An electrician might create a circuit with a short in it. A doctor might have a clear anatomical image. If you're a musician, perhaps you can see your pain as musical notes with discordant sounds. Create the image any way you like. Take your time. Details are the important thing. Now, fix it. Repair the damage you see using the best method possible for the mechanism you have created. The carpenter might replace the rotten wood or use epoxy to harden the rotten areas. The electrician will replace the circuit. The doctor will do surgery to fix the problem. The musician will rewrite the music. This might seem very simple but for me, it is very powerful and works every time. The key is to be very detailed in how you imagine the mechanism and take your time with it. Do not rush.

Breathing Through Your Fingertips

Let's try another of my favourite inductions: breathing through your fingertips.

You know how to start. Begin with breathing like always. In the remaining inductions I'll describe, I won't repeat this instruction because I know you understand the proper way to begin. For this induction you're going to do something a bit unusual. Imagine for a minute that you can actually breathe through your fingertips as opposed to through your mouth and nose. It's a little bit strange. Again, imagine just breathing through your fingertips.

Imagine that you can actually feel the air move up through the tips of your fingers, slowly into your fingers themselves. Let the air move into the deep tissues of your palm and fingers. Just take a deep breath into your hand and imagine it moving up through your fingertips. The air is moving in through your fingers and into the palms of your hands. Each time you breathe, you may be able to draw it up a little bit further, past your wrists, right up and through into your arms. Imagine the air flowing, flowing up, drawn up through fingertips, through your hands up through your arms and elbows. Draw the air higher and higher each time you breathe into your hand and draw the air up into your shoulders. The more deeply you breathe, the further you can pull this air up. Again starting from fingertips and pulling the air in, bring it up through your arms, past your shoulders, up your neck and into your head. Take deeper breaths now so you can pull it into your chest, down into your stomach. Perhaps the next breath can go into your legs. Deeper still and pull the air into your hands, your head, and down into your feet. You can feel the movement of the air throughout your body. It is an unusual idea to breathe through your fingertips but if you let yourself, you can actually feel the air move and each time it moves through, you allow yourself to become that much more relaxed. Everywhere the air touches inside the tension is relieved. More relaxed, less tense. You can feel the weight of your arms and legs lighten.

Pain Control Method

Now pay attention to an area that may be not as comfortable as some other part. Pick the easiest area first, not the one that's the worst, one that's just a little bit uncomfortable. Now move the air to that area and let the air soothe it. Let the air settle it down. The pain fades, becomes less intense. Breathe in. Less intense and less painful. Breathing in and breathing out. And if you are able to settle that area, try another area that might be a bit more uncomfortable. Focus on the air as you breathe it in through your fingertips. And just let it wash over the painful area. Just let it wash over it and let the pain fade. Just let the area fade away. Let the discomfort fade into the background. It becomes less important, not as interesting. It doesn't hold your attention as much. It is much more interesting to just feel the air moving in through your hands than to pay attention to the discomfort. If you're brave, pick some other area now that is that much more uncomfortable. See if you can move the relief from one area to this new painful area. Move the air in through your fingertips, up through your arms, into the area that you find uncomfortable. And as the air moves over it, the pain settles and dissipates. It becomes more distant perhaps. If it doesn't go away completely, it might just become less interesting. It recedes and doesn't hold your attention. It is less important. Remember you can return to this place the next time you do a trance. Remember where you are now.

Pain Control Method

While you're still in this trance, let's try another pain control method. Imagine that you have an injection of a local anaesthetic, lidocaine. It's similar to what is used by the dentist. When it's injected, you won't feel much of anything. It can be in a needle if you like. It can be in a super high-tech needle like on *Star Trek* where there is no needle. The liquid in the needle is injected by air pushing it through your skin. You can make up any device you want. Now you're going to use the injection on an area that's uncomfortable. If you can get relief, try it on another area.

When you're finished, bring yourself back.

Gloved-Hand Anaesthesia and the Candy Induction

Gloved-hand anaesthesia is a hypnotic phenomenon. I remember the first time I saw it demonstrated. I was in Washington DC, working with Dr. Nolan Bailey, who at the time was considered the hypnotists' hypnotist. He was working with a woman who was in my group. I remember that her entire arm became numb. He then had her transfer the feeling to her face, and she was shocked because according to her she felt like someone had given her an injection of local anaesthetic into her jaw. At the time, it was quite impressive. If you're able to create this phenomenon you're very fortunate. You can then transfer the feeling of anaesthesia from your hand to wherever you choose. You can do this by physically moving your arm and touching another area, or doing it in your mind's eye. I prefer having patients actually touch the area that they want to anaesthetize, but either method is fine. Let's get started.

Begin by breathing. Now use one of the inductions you already know—or perhaps you would like to try a new one that uses a different sensation. The one I'm going to describe uses the sense of taste. I call it the Candy Induction. Take a candy—it's best if it's a hard candy—you like the taste of. Now put it in your mouth and start the induction process by paying very close attention to the taste of the candy. Do not chew the candy or this will be over before you know it. Close your eyes. That's all you're going to do. Remember it's the internal banter that is important. I'm not going to do a complete banter script here—by now you should have a good feel for that. Take your time with this. Allow images time to come together. Give them as much detail as you can, using as many senses as you can. Now let's move to the next step.

Every time you get a good burst of taste out of the candy, associate it with a feeling of well-being. Associate it with something positive. Perhaps you get the image of something in your past, such as when you were small and were having something sweet like ice cream or candy cane. If you let it, candy can make you feel like a kid again. Not only is the taste of the candy associated with being a child again, but maybe with when you felt great, before you had any physical problems. You can remember when you were a perfectly healthy child. As a child you could relax yourself very easily because you didn't have that much on your mind. Let yourself relax and keep tasting the candy. Each time there is more flavour, the image of being young, healthy, and relaxed becomes stronger. Every taste lets you recall when you had almost no worries and almost no responsibilities of any kind. You felt like you could do anything you wanted to. You can remember when you had endless energy and you could go outside and play for hours and hours. Just let yourself relax and let the tension go. See if you can call up an image of a time when everything felt almost perfect for you. Perhaps you were with your family or on your own playing outside. Whatever that image is, give it as much substance as you can. Detail, detail, detail. Feel free to use the image you created before when you were relaxing if you prefer. Remember you can return to this place very easily—just start by tasting the same candy again. Once you have yourself in a good relaxed state, let's move on to gloved-hand anaesthesia.

Take a moment to look at your hands. Think about them for a moment and decide if one feels a bit different than the other one. Pick one. Left or right, it doesn't make a difference. Now that you've picked a hand, look at the back of it and notice if there is any area on the back that feels a bit different than the rest. If you find an area like that, put the index finger of your other hand over that area. If you can't feel a difference, then simply choose a spot on the back of your hand and let the opposite index finger rest on that spot. Once you have your finger on that spot, lift it up—touch and then stop touching that small area. Notice the difference between the feeling of touching and not touching. Or the difference between touch and release. Now do the same thing again, but see if, as you touch that area, you can make the feeling of touch recede. Make it go away so it feels the same as if you're not touching that small area. To test this, lift your finger up and let it drop down again on your hand. Notice the difference. With each touch down, the sensation becomes less and less. Lift your finger up and touch it down to your hand again—the sensation recedes. It becomes less and less. It is possible that the sensation recedes all at once. Or the sensation recedes bit by bit so it begins where sensation is reduced on the outside edge of a quarter-size part of your hand. As you tap down, that area increases until there is only a dime-size area with sensation and then that area gets progressively smaller until the entire quarter-size area has no sensation. Now let that area of numbness expand. Let it expand over the back of your hand. Let it spread over the knuckles. Always pay attention to the difference between the area of numbness and the other areas of your hand. Notice the difference between the back and palm of the hand. Now let the numb sensation spread around to the palm of your hand. Feel the difference between your hands. One might feel numb while the other does not. Continue to allow yourself to have the sensation in your hand recede. Perhaps the first time you do this there is only a minor difference. But the next time it will become more pronounced, and if you keep practising you might be able to numb your hand. You can use imagery to help with this process. One image is imagining you have ice on the back of the hand that moves to different parts of the hand, making it feel numb.

If you're able to create a sensation of numbness, the next step is to try to transfer that sensation. The first place is hand to hand. Clasp your hands together and allow the lack of sensation to move to the other hand. Again, imagery can be used to accomplish this. Perhaps the numbness is like radiant heat and you can see and feel a warm wave move from the numb hand to the other hand until both hands feel numb. If you can do this, you can move the feeling of numbness anywhere you want.

Let's try an example. If you have a painful back, take the numb hand and place it on your back. In your mind's eye, let the numbness move into your back. Spreading out and making the area feel numb. You might be able to use imagery to reinforce this. Two images come to my mind. The first is the most common image I use. I imagine I'm lying on a slab of ice. My back is resting on the ice. I can feel the cold moving into my back. I can see the ice melting because of the heat of my body but there is an endless amount of ice. It is sunny outside in my image but very cold and I'm just relaxing on a slab of ice that is now formed in the shape of my back. Sometimes when I do this, I actually shiver. If you've been able to transfer the numb feeling from your hand to your back, that's amazing. Now imagine that as you do that you can smell a scent or odour that's often associated with something that's cold and is often used to relax muscles. Can you smell menthol or eucalyptus? They have very distinct smells. See if you can smell those aromas—the stronger the smell, the deeper the numbness as it transfers to your back.

When you're finished, use a reversing technique. You know how to do this already.

Arm Levitation

Arm levitation—or the opposite, making an arm feel like it's made of lead—is a classic hypnotic induction. It forms the basis on which a stage hypnotist can select a subject, and it can give a person an idea of how suggestible they are, assuming that they don't "cheat" in the process. I'm showing it to you here because it's fun and has a link to stage hypnosis. I will include a pain control method as well. Let's begin.

Again, start with breathing, and when you're ready, close your eyes. Let both your arms rest on your lap or, if your chair has them, armrests. Breathe in and breathe out. Relax. If you don't want to close your eyes, simply use an eye fixation method and find a spot on a wall to look at and stay focused on that spot. With each breath in and each breath out, just let yourself feel more relaxed. Just let tension breathe out as you exhale. You can now pay attention to your hands and arms. Notice that one feels different than the other. Just a little different than the other hand. Just breathing in and out. Maybe you can feel a desire for the hand or arm to even move a little bit. Resist the temptation for now. Really pay attention and try to notice if one hand/arm feels lighter or heavier than the other. If not, take your time with it until you can get a sense of a difference like that. One arm might be more muscular. The Australian tennis player Rod Laver had the biggest right-left arm discrepancy I've ever seen. He would know right away which hand/arm is lighter and which is heavier. Once you feel the difference, let yourself enlarge the feeling. One hand is lighter than the other. As before, your hand or arm might want to move a bit, and if it does, you can let it move if you want. Let your arms and hands relax, starting at the fingertips and slowly moving up through the joints of the hand. Let the feeling spread across the palm of the hand over and around the back of the hand, breathing in. Almost as if you are breathing into your other hand and with each breath the hand and arm just become more relaxed. This is similar to breathing through your fingers, which you learned before. Now lift both arms out in front of you, palms up. Let your arms stay relaxed as you do this.

Now, on the arm that feels lighter, imagine that you have some helium balloons tied to that hand. Let's start with one balloon only. You can feel the pull of the helium-filled balloon on that hand/arm. On the heavier side, imagine a large dictionary book is put onto your palm. You can feel the weight. So, one side has a pull upward and you can feel your arm being pulled up, while the other side is being pushed down by the weight of the book. Pay attention to the differences between the two sides. One side feels progressively lighter while the other feels progressively heavier.

Now, if you want to you can amplify the feeling by tying another helium-filled balloon to the lighter hand/arm and put another heavy book onto the hand on the other side. One side is being pulled upward and feels very light while the other has a tremendous weight on it and is being pulled down. You can now put as many balloons as you want to on the light side and as many heavy books as you would like on the heavy side. Imagine how that feels. Allow yourself to feel it. Feel the pull up and the push down. Feel one arm being pulled up and up while the other is pushed down further and further.

Now, let yourself open your eyes but at the same time maintain a sense of "trance." Keep yourself relaxed. Or you can have someone else observe you at this point. What do you see? Is one arm up while the other is down? Is the movement just a bit or none at all? If you see a difference, that is evidence of suggestibility. A stage hypnotist would build on this finding to make sure that you are the right person to be hypnotized on stage. If you have a big difference between the two sides, that's a great start for stage hypnosis. But you're going to use it for a different purpose.

Close your eyes again and let yourself relax. Keep the balloons attached to your arm but you can let go of those heavy books if you like. Focus on the arm with the balloons.

Feel the tug upward. Breathe in and out. Use one of our deepening exercises or make one up yourself. I scuba dive so I use an image of scuba diving to deepen my trance.

Pain Control Method

Now, find an uncomfortable sensation inside of you. Locate it. Now see if you can move it into one of those balloons. Imagine your discomfort moving from where it usually is, through your body, down your arm, and into a balloon. Once you have the image, release that balloon. Let it go. Let it float upward, and as it does, it takes your pain with it. As it floats away, you let yourself forget about that particular pain. Let the balloon keep floating until it disappears. Let the pain go with it. Let it disappear. If you are successful, pick another area of discomfort and do the same thing, floating the feeling away. You can do this as many times as you like, as long as you're getting an effect. If not, stop and practise until you can get the effect. When you're finished doing this trance, bring yourself back using proper methods.

Ring Induction

I am now going to do something counterintuitive. This is a method used in hypnosis to work with people who simply cannot relax. I say "Relax" and they get tense. I remember using this method on a very big body builder. He had the biggest, tenses muscles I've ever seen. Relaxing was something he simply did not understand and the idea of it made him nervous. I'm going to mix this induction with another induction method that people in my group programs enjoy.

If you have a ring, great. Make sure it is on a finger that you can easily look at. If you don't have a ring, no problem, make it out of a bit of tin foil. Now start by simply looking at the ring.

You know how to do this already. Rather than using a wall, we're simply using the ring. You can use either the eyelid induction while focusing on the ring or some of the basics you've learned. Keep looking at the ring and as you do, allow yourself to become progressively more tense. That's right ... tense. Start at the top of your head and search out each muscle, one by one and when you find it, tense it. The only caveat is, if you have an area of pain, leave that alone. Do not tense those muscles. The object here is to increase your body's tension, not pain. Keep going. Search out muscles in your neck and outward to your shoulders. Tense the muscles. Tense for as long as you can without causing pain and then let go. If the muscle is not too fatigued, tense it again and let go. Move from area to area, slowly. Across your shoulders and into your arms and hands. Down your neck to your chest, stomach, and around to the back. Tensing and releasing as you go. Now down your legs and ending in your feet. Tense, relax. Tense, relax. Now simply let all of it go. Let yourself go. You are now in a perfect position to do a deepening exercise. Use one of mine or your own.

Now take a moment to check out the pain in your body. Find an area that's uncomfortable. Earlier, you gave it colour and a number. Now imagine that the pain is a musical sound from a record or CD. You can imagine playing it. You can hear it very clearly. It might be discordant symphonic music or it can be independent sounds that are not musical at all. Imagine that the sound is emanating from the record or CD. Now, in your mind's eye turn down the sound. Your player has a very large volume knob. You can't miss it. You're slowly turning the knob, and as you do, the pain starts to recede. Note by note, sound by sound, it recedes as you turn it down. You can hear it less and less, and as that happens you feel it less and less. Take your time with this one. Once you have done this with one area of discomfort, move on to another area and repeat the procedure. Take your time. If it doesn't work the first time, don't worry. Keep practising and you'll get there eventually. Once you're ready, bring yourself back.

Sitting to Standing

You might recall that I've mentioned that eventually you want to be able to use these methods when you're active. That's why I don't start from a lying-down position. You start sitting. Once you've mastered the method and understand how to induce a simple trance for pain control, the next step is inducing a trance in a less favourable condition. You don't have to go from sitting to running. Instead you can work from sitting still but perhaps learn how to induce a trance while the room is noisy or there are people around you doing things. Eventually you will go from sitting to standing, learning how to induce a trance while standing in a protected environment like your home. Once you have that mastered, you can take the method on the road. Find a place to go to that isn't too noisy or busy and see if you can induce a trance in that setting. If you can't, come back and try again and again. Eventually you will get it. Now try your hand at a busier environment. Keep going until you're able to do it while standing in a moving subway. After all these years, I can do it anywhere—and remember, I'm not a good subject.

Sleep

The methods I've described are excellent for sleep induction. What you want to do is pick one or two simple ones. If you use them for sleep, though, don't use them for pain control. Just use them for sleep. I often add physical movement to the induction because it's hard for me to shut off my thinking. I find that if I add a bit of movement, it stops my thinking. By way of example, while I'm lying down I'll use one finger from my right hand to trace out a letter from the alphabet on my leg or arm or whatever part is nearby and easy to access. After I trace out the letter, I then use my entire hand and erase it. After A, I then trace B and so on. If I make a mistake, I return to the beginning. If I get distracted and forget where I was, I start over. If I finish the alphabet, I start over. This will usually work for me within three rounds of going through the alphabet.

In this chapter I've described a variety of methods of induction and pain control. What I've outlined is the basis for the 10-week treatment program at my clinic. If you practise and can get a handle on this tool, your pain should be more manageable. The most important thing to remember is that you have to practise over and over again in order to make hypnosis useful.

Conclusion

B y reading through this book and practising the inductions, you will know more about self-hypnosis for pain
control than almost any physician or person you will see
in your lifetime. By practising, you will become an expert.

I hope that you can see why self-hypnosis for pain control
should play a role in the management of chronic pain for
patients. Although medications can help, they don't help
everyone and they all carry potential side effects, some more
serious than others. In the case of opioids, the most commonly used analgesic for chronic pain, the worst possible
side effects include addiction to the medication and even
death. Even if these terrible side effects do not occur, their
efficacy is limited. Self-hypnosis, on the other hand, is a
potentially effective method of pain control that causes no
harm and, once learned, has no cost. What could be better!

One of the primary limiting factors preventing patients from learning self-hypnosis for pain control is that very few clinicians know how to do it. It is not part of their typical training. It was never mentioned throughout all my training, both as a medical student and as a resident in psychiatry. This might be because the association with stage hypnosis has tarnished its reputation in medical circles. As I've explained, clinical hypnosis is not stage hypnosis. It is a very different skill set with a very different purpose. It is not for entertainment. It is to help people.

Hopefully, with time, clinical hypnosis will become recognized as a useful tool to help patients with chronic pain. When this happens, more training opportunities will develop and more clinicians will learn the skill and more patients will have the potential to be helped safely.

If you decide that you want to go to a hypnotherapist to learn more skills for pain control, it is important that you make sure they can deliver the goods. That's not easy, even for someone like me. Recently I decided to update my training in hypnotherapy, so I contacted many hypnotherapists from around the world. Out of 20 therapists, only one had any real clinical designation. The reason I chose not to train with him is that he worked in a very specific form of hypnotherapy and treated it more like a religion than a method of helping people. Like I've said, to date, no research has been done that proves one method of self-hypnosis is better than another. For me hypnotherapy is a treatment, not a religion, so I scratched him from my list. A number of others disappeared once they found out I was a psychiatrist with years of practice in teaching self-hypnosis. The rest came across as people who probably did stage hypnosis and moved into clinical hypnosis because they found it more lucrative. You have to be careful. You want to find a clinician who is dedicated to helping people.

The best way to do that is to find someone who has a clinical qualification like a physician, a psychologist, a nurse, or a social worker. Talk to them first. Find out what method of treatment they use and if they see it as a tool to help others or a religion that should not be tampered with. Next, find out what they understand about chronic pain and how many other people they have treated with your type of problem. If possible, see if you can get a reference. This can be difficult because they cannot give you the name of a patient, unless that patient agrees, because of confidentiality. I have a patient who has agreed to talk to any patient with questions. He is very open and honest.

Good luck with your search if this is the direction you take. But appreciate that in your hands you hold the method of teaching self-hypnosis that I have used for over 30 years. Practise, practise, practise and use your skill in moving from the outside-in to gain control of your chronic pain.

Appendix: Acupressure Induction

As you've seen, there are a multitude of different inductions, and, as I've said before, there is no evidence that one works better than another. Find the ones you like. This induction is a bit more complex because it is a mix of acupressure and hypnosis. In my group program, patients really enjoy this one.

This induction combines using classic acupressure points with hypnosis. Acupunture, which uses very fine needles inserted at those points, has been around for thousands of years as a method to relieve pain, among other things. Acupressure uses finger pressure instead of needles. When you practise acupressure, you don't want to put so much pressure that you leave bruising; as well, don't use your nail or anything sharp, just your fingertip. Certain acupuncture points are associated with putting a person in a more relaxed state and others are used to control pain. Let's see how we can use these while doing hypnosis.

Acupuncture points have names based on acupuncture meridians. These meridians occur all over the body—but they have nothing to do with Western medicine and, in fact, make no sense at all to a Western physician. For example, one of the lines is called the kidney line or the great intestine line, but it has nothing to do with the anatomical placement of the kidney. The meridian is nowhere near where the kidney is and these lines are certainly not where the great intestine is. But the theory of these lines was developed a long time ago and the practice based on this theory has been used for thousands of years.

Before we get too far, there is one important question to ask. Does acupuncture work? I ask about acupuncture not pressure, because there is a lot more literature about acupuncture. The long and short of it is that there is evidence that acupuncture works for certain problems like migraines, neck disorders, tension-type headaches, and peripheral joint osteoarthritis. At this point, the evidence is considered inconclusive for shoulder pain, lateral elbow pain, and low back pain. So based on this evidence, let's begin.

There are four powerful energy points in acupuncture. They are Stomach (ST36) or the Leg Three Miles or Zusanii Point; Large Intestine (LI4) or the He Gu or Hoku point (it means Union Valley); Liver (LV3 or LR3) point or Tai Chong or Great Surge point; and the Spleen (SP6) point or San Yin Jiao Point. Let's take them one by one. The letters in the name stand for the meridian that the point is on and the number is the point's specific location. The scientist in me feels compelled to tell you there is no great scientific evidence for most of the claims associated with these points. Nonetheless acupuncture is an ancient art and who knows, maybe the originators got it right.

The first point we're going to use is ST36. ST36 is thought to help with chronic illness, nausea, vomiting, depression, nervousness, and overall well-being, as well as improve longevity. ST36 is located four finger widths

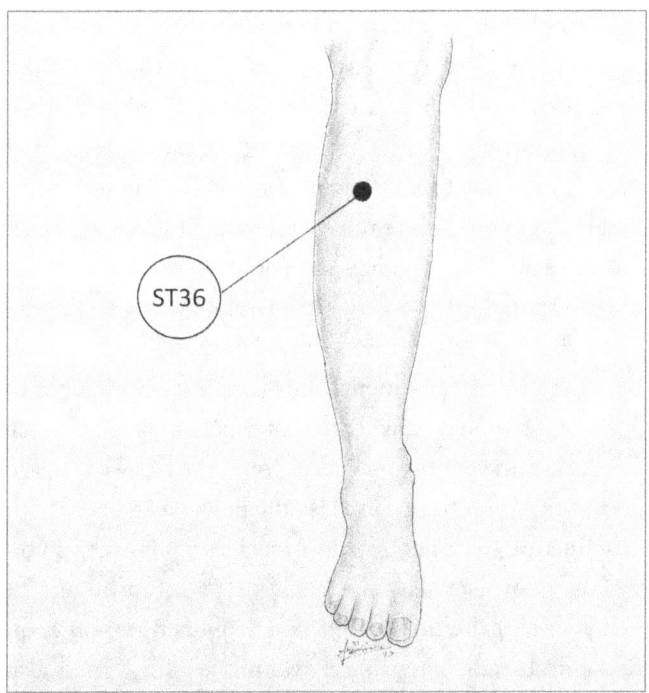

(cun) down from the bottom of your knee cap. Now move along the outer boundary of your shin bone. If you are in the right place, a muscle can be felt under your finger as you move your foot up and down.

Now place your finger on ST36. You can use both sides or just one side—it makes no difference, just do what is physically comfortable. You are now touching a major energy point. If you want, close your eyes and just put some pressure on that point. It should be a bit uncomfortable. Acupuncturists will tell you that if you're on the right point it should hurt a bit. The pressure you use should not be painful. Don't try to drill through to the other side of your leg. As you put pressure on ST36, use some of the skills you already know. Start box breathing or bumble bee breathing. If you want, you can use the simple breathing induction of five breaths in and out and then hold for five breaths. Or you can use the eyelid induction. As you "turn on" this acupressure point, see if you can feel a deeper sense of relaxation. As you do any of the inductions, also keep in mind that you're stirring up a major energy point in the body. Try to create a mental image of energy changes in your body as you do this. Take your time. Put detail into the image. Let the energy permeate your body. Move it to the areas where you have pain. Use the power associated with acupuncture to settle the pain. Now let's try another point.

This point is a "big one." It is Large Intestine or LI4 and is one of the most important acupuncture points on the body. It is the big pain reliever of the body. This is also

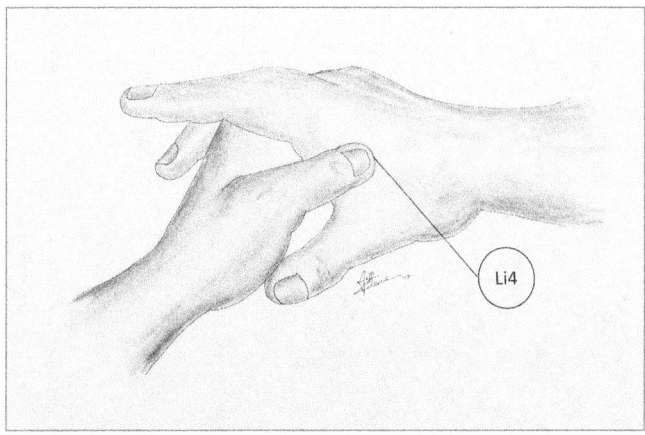

called the Hoku point. It is located on the back of the hand, in the webbing where the thumb and index finger meet. To find the exact point, bring your thumb and index finger together. The muscle will bulge a little and that is the spot. I have never met an acupuncturist who does not activate LI4 in any treatment session. Again, repeat the procedure. Use a breathing technique of simple trance. Let yourself relax. Activate LI4. Create an image of how the Hoku point might actually relieve pain in the body. Get into it. Use your breathing to relax your body (or another induction you have decided to use) and allow your imagination to take the power of the Hoku and spread it throughout your body. Use it to control areas of pain. That is one of the primary purposes of this point.

Next is LV3, a reflection of the Hoku point but in the foot. This point is on the top of the foot between the big

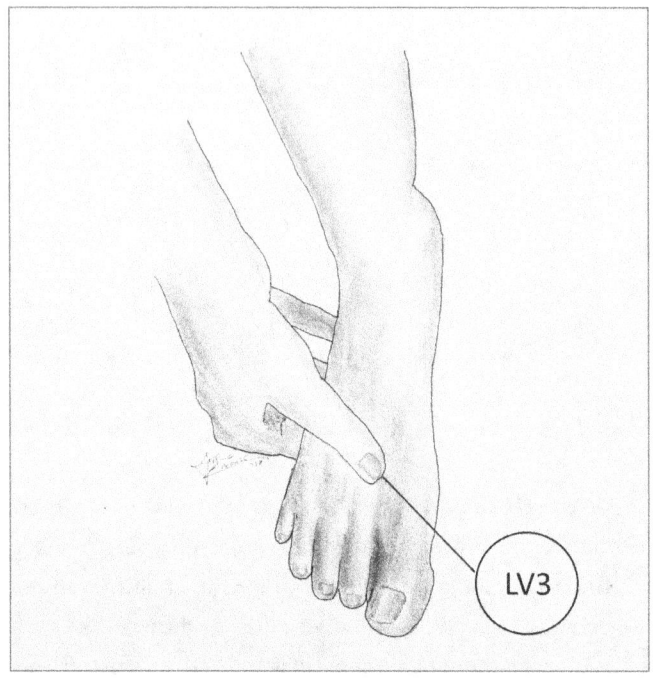

toe and the second toe. It is just like the Hoku point but it's on your foot instead of on your hand. It is also a powerful point. It can help with anger, irritability, insomnia, and anxiety. It is used for eye problems and digestive problems. Put this together with the Hoku point and you can have a huge impact on energy flow in the body. Try using this point by itself, then add the Hoku point at the same time and see if there is a difference for you. Do the same thing you've done so far: Use breathing or a simple induction. Relax. Create an image of the movement of energy as you activate the point. Take your time with this. Allow the point to decrease your pain and improve your level of energy.

The last point of the four energy points is SP6. This point is located on the inside of your leg, just above your ankle. To find this point, locate the highest point of your ankle. From this point, move four finger widths up your leg. This is where the point is located. There is a precaution for this point. The San Yin Jiao (SP6) should not be used in pregnancy because this point is thought to induce labour. Activating it can also can help with sexual function in men. Again, do the same thing as you have done with the other three points.

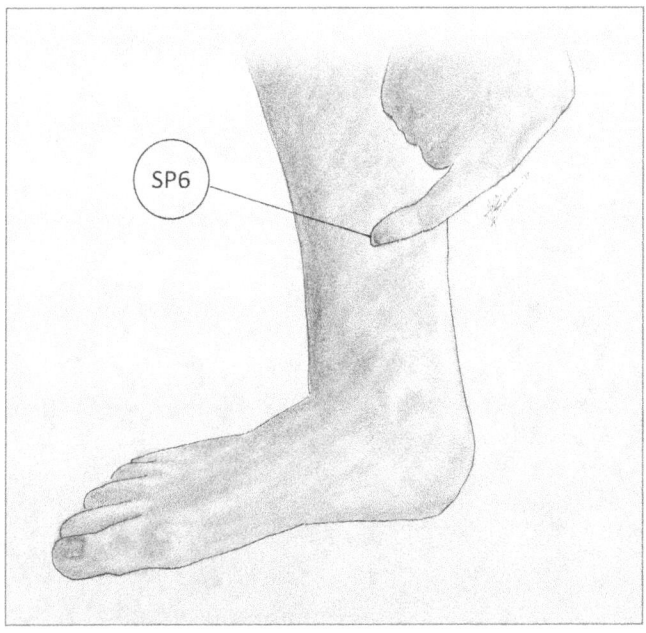

If you find this type of treatment helpful, go online to find more acupuncture points to try. I have selected the four powerful energy points of acupuncture but there are hundreds of other points to try. Enjoy experimenting.

Relevant Websites

D r. Ennis, along with Gilda, has set up endowment funds across Canada. These endowment funds are located at McMaster University in Hamilton, Ontario; University of Toronto in Toronto, Ontario; and the University of British Columbia in Vancouver, British Columbia. Money from the endowment funds is awarded to a deserving resident each year who shows an interest in helping patients with chronic pain. The money is used to further the resident's education in the field of chronic pain, with the goal of helping develop new pain specialists. Donate to the endowment fund through the following website:

www.ennisendowment.com

Dr. Ennis has made his artwork available for sale. All profits from these sales go to the Ennis Endowment Fund. You can find his work at:

www.ennisendowmentfund.com

Dr. Ennis, along with Richard Waterhouse, has developed the Hypnotherapy for Pain Control App. It is designed to augment this book. The inductions are done by Dr. Ennis and some of the clinicians who work in his clinic. These are the same inductions used in Dr. Ennis's hypnotherapy program. Like this book, part of the proceeds from the sale of the app goes to the Ennis Endowment Fund. The app can be found at:

www.hypnotherapyforpaincontrol.com

References

Introduction

http://nationalpaincentre.mcmaster.ca/documents/Opioid%20GL%20
for%20CMAJ_01may2017.pdf

3 What You Need to Know About Chronic Pain

Bennett GJ. Update on the neurophysiology of pain transmission and modulation: focus on the NMDA-receptor. *J Pain Symptom Manage*. 2000 Jan; 19(1 Suppl):S2–6.

Bolay H, Moskowitz MA. Mechanisms of pain modulation in chronic syndromes. *Neurology*. 2002; 59(5 Suppl 2):S2–S7.

Borsook D. A future without chronic pain: neuroscience and clinical research. *Cerebrum*. 2012 May/June. [Epub 2012 Jun 27].

Borsook D, Sava S, Becerra L. The pain imaging revolution: advancing pain into the 21st century. *Neuroscientist*. 2010;16:171–185.

Fishman SM. "Pain as the fifth vital sign: how can I tell when back pain is serious." *Journal of Pain & Palliative Care Pharmacotherapy*. Vol. 19, No. 4, 2005, pp. 77–79.

Gold MS, Gebhart GF. Nociceptor sensitization in pain pathogenesis. *Nature Medicine*. 2010; 16(11): 1248–1257.

Henry DE, Chiodo AE, Yang W. Central nervous system reorganization in a variety of chronic pain states: a review. *PM R*. 2011;3:1116–1125.

Herrero JF, Laird JM, López-García JA. Wind-up of spinal cord neurones and pain sensation: much ado about something? *ProgNeurobiol*. 2000;61(2):169–203.

Kuner R. Central mechanisms of pathological pain. *Nature Medicine*. 2010;16(11):1258–1266.

Latremoliere A, Woolf CJ. Central Sensitization: A Generator of Pain Hypersensitivity by Central Neural Plasticity. *J Pain*. 2009 Sep;10(9):895–926.

Schopflocher D, Taenzer P, Jovey R. The prevalence of chronic pain in Canada. *Pain Res Manag*. 2011 Nov–Dec;16(6): 445–450.

Schweinhardt P, Bushnell MC. Pain imaging in health and disease— how far have we come? *J Clin Invest*. 2010;120:3788–3797.

4   The Problem With Pills

Andreae MH, Carter GM, Shaparin N, Suslov K, Ellis RJ, Ware MA, Abrams DI, Prasad H, Wilsey B, Indyk D, Johnson M9, Sacks HS. Inhaled cannabis for chronic neuropathic pain: a meta-analysis of individual patient data. *J Pain*. 2015 Dec;16(12):1221–1232.

Ballantyne, J, Shin, NS. Efficacy of opioids for chronic pain: a review of the evidence. *Clinical Journal of Pain*. 2008;24:469–478.

Centers for Disease Control and Prevention. CDC guideline for prescribing opioids for chronic pain—United States. *Morbidity and Mortality Weekly Report*. 2016 May 15.

Chou R, Peterson K, Helfand M. Comparative efficacy and safety of skeletal muscle relaxants for spasticity and musculoskeletal conditions: a systematic review. *Journal of Pain and Symptom Management*. 2004;28(2):140–175.

Chou R, Turner JA, Devine EB, Hansen RN, Sullivan SD, Blazina I, Dana T, Bougatsos C, Deyo RA. The effectiveness and risks of long-term opioid therapy for chronic pain: a systematic review for a National Institutes of Health Pathways to Prevention Workshop. *Ann Intern Med*. 2015 Feb 17;162(4):276–286.

Cohen SP, Christo PJ, Wang S, Chen L, Stojanovic MP, Shields CH, Brummett C, Mao J. The effect of opioid dose and treatment duration on the perception of a painful standardized clinical stimulus. *Reg Anesth Pain Med*. 2008 May–Jun;33(3):199–206.

Collen M. Opioid contracts and random drug testing for people with chronic pain—think twice. *The Journal of Law, Medicine & Ethics*. 2009;37(4):841–845.

Davies NM, Jamali F. COX-2 selective inhibitors cardiac toxicity: getting to the heart of the matter. *J Pharm PharmaceutSci*. 2004;7(3):332–336.

De Maddalena C, Bellini M, Berra M, Meriggiola MC, Aloisi AM. Opioid-induced hypogonadism: why and how to treat it. *Pain Physician*. 2012 Jul;15(3 Suppl):ES111–118.

Drug Testing: *A bad investment*. American Civil Liberties Union. 1999.

Eriksen J, Sjøgren P, Bruera E, Ekholm O, Rasmussen NK. Critical issues on opioids in chronic non-cancer pain: an epidemiological study. *Pain*. 2006;125(1-2): 172–179.

Gabapentin for chronic neuropathic pain and fibromyalgia in adults. *Cochrane Database for Systematic Reviews*. 2015.

Giardiello FM. NSAID-induced polyp regression in familial adenomatous polyposis patients. *GastroenterolClin North Am*. 1996 Jun;25(2):349–362.

Hamid S, Yakoob J, Jafri W, Islam S, Abid S, Islam M. Frequency of NSAID induced peptic ulcer disease. *J Pak Med Assoc.* 2006 May;56(5):218–222.

Honarmand A, Safavi M, Zare M. *Gabapentin: An update of its pharmacological properties and therapeutic use in epilepsy.* J Res Med Sci. 2011 Aug; 16(8): 1062–1069.

Kroenke K, Krebs EE, Bair MJ. Pharmacotherapy of chronic pain: a synthesis of recommendations from systematic reviews. *General Hospital Psychiatry.* 2009 May–June;(31)3:206–219.

Marconi A, Di Forti M, Lewis CM, Murray RM, Vassos E. Meta-analysis of the association between the level of cannabis use and risk of psychosis. *Schizophr Bull.* 2016 Sep;42(5):1262–1269.

Moore RA, Straube S, Wiffen PJ, Derry S, McQuay HJ. Pregabalin for acute and chronic pain in adults. *Cochrane Database Syst Rev.* 2009 Jul 8;(3):CD007076.

Schiltenwolf M, Akbar M, Hug A, Pfüller U, Gantz S, Neubauer E, Flor H, Wang H. Evidence of specific cognitive deficits in patients with chronic low back pain under long-term substitution treatment of opioids. *Pain Physician.* 2014 Jan–Feb;17(1):9–20.

Starrels JL, Becker WC, Alford DP, Kapoor A, Williams AR, Turner BJ. Systematic review: treatment agreements and urine drug testing to reduce opioid misuse in patients with chronic pain. *Ann Intern Med.* 2010 Jun 1;152(11):712–720.

Teater D. Evidence for efficacy of pain medications. National Saftety Council (Manuscript). Nd.

Trescot A, Glaser SE, Hansen H, Benyamin R, Patel S, Manchikanti L. Effectiveness of opioids in the treatment of chronic non-cancer pain. *Pain Physician.* 2008; 11(2 Suppl): S181–200.

Wang R, Huanag PC. Patent protection of pharmacologically active metabolites: theoretical and technological analysis on the jurisprudence of four regions. *Santa Clara High Technology Law Journal*. 2012;29(3): 489–521.

Ware MA, Gamsa A, Persson J, Fitzcharles MA. Cannabis for chronic pain: case series and implications for clinicians. *Pain Res Manag*. 2002 Summer;7(2):95–99.

Ware MA, Wang T, Shapiro S, Robinson A, Ducruet T, Huynh T, Gamsa A, Bennett GJ, Collet JP. Smoked cannabis for chronic neuropathic pain: a randomized controlled trial. *CMAJ*. 2010 Oct 5;182(14):E694–701.

Zhang LR, Morgenstern H, Greenland S, Chang SC, Lazarus P, Teare MD, Woll PJ, Orlow I, Cox B, Cannabis and Respiratory Disease Research Group of New Zealand, Brhane Y, Liu G, Hung RJ. Cannabis smoking and lung cancer risk: pooled analysis in the International Lung Cancer Consortium. *Int J Cancer*. 2015 Feb 15;136(4):894–903.

6   History of Hypnosis

Donaldson IML. Mesmer's 1780 proposal for a controlled trial to test his method of treatment using "animal magnetism." *J R Soc Med*. 2005 Dec; 98(12): 572–575

7   The Science Behind Hypnosis: Does It Work? How?

Accardi MC, Milling LS. The effectiveness of hypnosis for reducing procedure-related pain in children and adolescents: a comprehensive methodological review. *Journal of Behavioral Medicine*. 2009;32: 328–339.

Adachi T, Fujino H, Nakae A, Mashimo T, Sasaki J. A meta-analysis of hypnosis for chronic pain problems. *Intl. Journal of Clinical and Experimental Hypnosis*. 2014;62(1):1–28.

Avenanti A, Minio-Paluello I, Bufalari I, Aglioti SM. The pain of a model in the personality of an onlooker. *NeuroImage*. 2009;44(1):275–283.

Barber J, Mayer D. Evaluation of the efficacy and neural mechanism of a hypnotic analgesia procedure in experimental and clinical dental pain. *Pain*. 1977;4:41–48.

Cojan Y, Piguet C, Vuilleumier P. What makes your brain suggestible? hypnotizability is associated with differential brain activity during attention outside hypnosis. *NeuroImage*. 2015:117:367–374.

Cramer H, Lauche R, Paul A, Langhorst J, Kümmel S, Dobos GJ. Integrative cancer therapies. 2015;14(1):5–15.

De Pascalis V, Magurano MR, Bellusci A, Chen AC. Somatosensory event-related potential and autonomic activity to varying pain reduction cognitive strategies in hypnosis. *Clinical Neurophysiology*. 2001;112:1475–1485.

Derbyshire SW, Whalley MG, Stenger VA, Oakley DA. Cerebral activation during hypnotically induced and imagined pain. *NeuroImage*. 2004;23:392–401.

Dienes Z., Perner J. 2007. The cold control theory of hypnosis. In G. Jamieson (Ed.), *Hypnosis and Conscious States: The Cognitive Neuroscience Perspective*. Oxford: Oxford University Press, 293–314.

Donaldson IML. Mesmer's 1780 proposal for a controlled trial to test his method of treatment using "animal magnetism." *J R Soc Med*. 2005 Dec; 98(12): 572–575.

Gruzeler J. H. A working model of the neurophysiology of hypnosis: a review of evidence. *Contemporary Hypnosis*. 1998;15:3–21.

Halligan PW, Athwal BS, Oakley DA, Frackowiak RSJ. The functional anatomy of a hypnotic paralysis: implications for conversion hysteria. *The Lancet*. 2000;356:986–987.

Hilgard ER. 1977. *Divided Consciousness: Multiple Controls in Human Thought and Action*. New York, NY: Wiley.

Kihlstrom JF. 2008. The doman of hypnosis revisited. In M. R. Nash & A. J. Barnier (eds). *The Oxford Handbook of Hypnosis: Theory, Research and Practice*. Oxford: Oxford University Press.

Kirjanen S. Brain activity during pain relief using hypnosis and placebo treatments: a literature review. *Journal of European Psychology Students*. 2012;3:78–87.

Kirsch I, Lynn SJ. Hypnotic involuntariness and the automaticity of everyday life. *American Journal of Clinical Hypnosis*. 1997;40:329–348.

Levine JD, Gordon NC, Fields HL. The mechanisms of placebo analgesia. *Lancet*. 1978;2:654–657.

Mazzoni G, Venneri A, McGeown WJ, Kirsch I. Neuroimaging resolution of the altered state hypothesis. *Cortex*. 2013;49:400–410.

Oakley DA, Halligan PW. Hypnotic suggestion and cognitive neuroscience. *Trends in Cognitive Sciences*. 2009;13(6):264–270.

Page RA, Green JP. An update on age, hypnotic suggestibility, and gender: a brief report. *American Journal of Clinical Hypnosis*. 2007;49(4):283–287.

Patterson DR, Jensen MP. Hypnosis and clinical pain. *Psychological Bulletin*. 2003;129(4):495–521.

Spanos NP, Menary E, Gabora NJ, DuBreuil SC, Dewhirst B. Secondary identity enactments during hypnotic past-life regression: a sociocognitive perspective. *Journal of Personality and Social Psychology*. 1991;61:308–320.

Vanhaudenhuyse A, Laureys S, Faymonville ME. Neurophysiology of hypnosis. *Clinical Neurophysiology*. 2014;44:343–353.

9   Outside In: How to Hypnotize Yourself for Pain Relief

Kabat-Zinn J. An outpatient program in behavioral medicine for chronic pain patients based on the practice of mindfulness meditation: theoretical considerations and preliminary results. *Gen Hosp Psychiatry*. 1982 Apr;4(1):33–47.

Damush TM, Kroenke K, Bair MJ, Wu J, Tu W, Krebs E, Poleshuck E. Pain self-management training increases self-efficacy, self-management behaviours and pain and depression outcomes. *Eur J Pain*. 2016;15:213–219.

Appendix: Acupressure Induction

Lee MS, Ernst E. Acupuncture for pain: an overview of Cochrane reviews. *Chin J Integr Med*. 2011 Mar;17(3):187–189.

About the Author

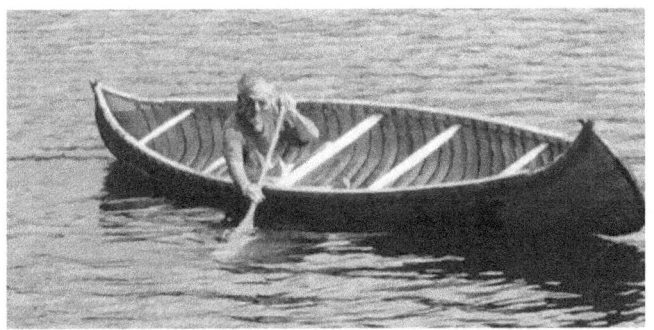

D r. Jeffrey Ennis is a world-class expert in managing chronic non-cancer pain. Trained as a psychiatrist, he is the medical director of the Ennis Centre for Pain Management in Hamilton, and an assistant clinical professor with the Department of Rehabilitation Medicine, the Department of Psychiatry and Behavioural Neurosciences at McMaster University Medical Centre. He's also a clinical instructor at the University of British Columbia Department of Psychiatry. He lectures on chronic pain management at medical conferences across Canada and in Europe.

www.ingramcontent.com/pod-product-compliance
Lightning Source LLC
Chambersburg PA
CBHW051308220526
45468CB00004B/1252